The DMSO Healing Solution

A Step-by-Step Guide to Safely Harnessing Dimethyl Sulfoxide for Effective Pain Relief, Inflammation Reduction, and Chronic Condition Management

Evelyn Sinclair

Table of Contents

Introduction

What Is DMSO?

Dimethyl sulfoxide (DMSO) is an organosulfur compound with the molecular formula $(CH_3)_2SO$. It is a colorless, odorless liquid at room temperature and is characterized by its remarkable ability to dissolve both polar and nonpolar compounds, making it a versatile solvent in chemical and pharmaceutical industries. DMSO is hygroscopic, meaning it readily absorbs water from the atmosphere, and is miscible with a wide range of organic solvents and water.

Chemically, DMSO is classified as a **polar aprotic solvent**. This classification indicates that it has a high dielectric constant but lacks hydrogen atoms that can participate in hydrogen bonding with solutes. Its molecular structure consists of a sulfur atom double-bonded to an oxygen atom and single-bonded to two methyl groups. This unique arrangement imparts distinctive physicochemical properties, such as a high boiling point (189°C) and the ability to stabilize radical species.

DMSO is primarily derived from lignin, a major component of wood, as a byproduct of the paper manufacturing industry. Its industrial production involves the oxidation of dimethyl sulfide, another sulfur-containing compound, using oxygen or nitrogen dioxide as oxidants.

In biological contexts, DMSO is renowned for its exceptional ability to penetrate biological membranes without causing significant damage. This permeability facilitates its use as a carrier molecule for delivering pharmaceuticals transdermally. Additionally, DMSO exhibits anti-inflammatory, analgesic, and antioxidant properties, which have been the subject of extensive biomedical research.

From a pharmacological perspective, DMSO interacts with cellular components such as proteins and lipids. It can modulate enzyme activity, alter membrane fluidity, and affect the folding and aggregation of proteins. These interactions are concentration-dependent and can lead to varied biological effects, some of which are therapeutically beneficial.

In laboratory settings, DMSO is frequently used as a solvent for the storage and administration of small molecules in biological experiments. Its low toxicity to cells at appropriate concentrations makes it suitable for use in cell culture systems. Furthermore, DMSO is employed in cryopreservation protocols for cells and tissues due to its ability to protect biological structures from damage during freezing.

Despite its widespread use, DMSO is not without limitations. At higher concentrations, it can induce cytotoxic effects and disrupt cellular function. Therefore, careful consideration of dosing and exposure time is crucial in both experimental and therapeutic applications.

In summary, dimethyl sulfoxide is a chemically and biologically significant compound with a wide array of applications stemming from its unique molecular properties. Its role as a solvent, permeation enhancer, and bioactive molecule continues to make it a valuable subject of study in both scientific research and clinical practice.

History and Discovery of DMSO

The story of dimethyl sulfoxide (DMSO) begins in the mid-19th century with its initial synthesis by Russian chemist Alexander Zaytsev in 1866. While studying oxidation reactions of dimethyl sulfide, Zaytsev isolated DMSO as a byproduct. Despite this early discovery, DMSO remained a chemical curiosity for several decades, largely confined to laboratory settings without significant practical applications.

The compound's unique properties began to garner attention in the mid-20th century. In the 1950s, industrial chemists recognized DMSO's exceptional solvent capabilities, particularly its ability to dissolve both polar and nonpolar compounds. This dual solubility made it valuable in the petrochemical and polymer industries, where it was used to process and manufacture polymers, resins, and other complex materials.

A pivotal moment in DMSO's history occurred in the early 1960s when Dr. Stanley W. Jacob, a surgeon at the Oregon Health & Science University, initiated medical research into the compound. Dr. Jacob was investigating cryopreservation techniques and was intrigued by DMSO's ability to protect red blood cells and other biological tissues from damage during freezing. His experiments revealed that DMSO could penetrate biological membranes without causing cellular destruction, a property not commonly found in other solvents.

Dr. Jacob's research expanded to explore DMSO's potential therapeutic benefits. Preliminary studies suggested anti-inflammatory, analgesic, and diuretic effects, sparking interest in its application for conditions such as arthritis, musculoskeletal injuries, and scleroderma. The compound's ability to act as a carrier molecule also opened avenues for transdermal drug delivery, as it could transport pharmaceuticals across the skin barrier more efficiently.

In the mid-1960s, clinical trials were initiated to assess DMSO's efficacy and safety in humans. However, the path was not without obstacles. Reports of adverse effects, including changes in ocular lens refractive indices in animal studies, raised safety concerns. The U.S. Food and Drug Administration (FDA) imposed restrictions, halting some clinical trials to further evaluate potential risks.

Despite setbacks, research continued globally. In 1978, the FDA approved DMSO for the treatment of interstitial cystitis, a chronic inflammatory condition of the bladder. This approval marked the first official therapeutic use of DMSO in conventional medicine within the United States. Concurrently, other countries adopted DMSO for various medical applications, recognizing its therapeutic potential.

Throughout the latter half of the 20th century, DMSO's profile grew within alternative medicine circles. It was explored for off-label uses, including treatment for sprains, burns, and even as an adjunct therapy in cancer care. While anecdotal reports and preliminary studies indicated benefits, the lack of large-scale, controlled clinical trials limited widespread medical acceptance.

In addition to human medicine, DMSO found a place in veterinary practice. It was used to treat musculoskeletal disorders in horses and other animals, leveraging its anti-inflammatory and analgesic properties. The equine industry, in particular, embraced DMSO for conditions like laminitis and tendon injuries.

The late 20th and early 21st centuries saw advancements in understanding DMSO at the molecular level. Research delved into its mechanisms of action, exploring how DMSO interacts with water molecules, proteins, and cell membranes. These studies provided insights into its cryoprotective abilities and effects on cellular processes, informing safer and more effective use.

Despite ongoing debates regarding its applications, DMSO remains a compound of interest in both scientific research and clinical practice. Its journey from a simple chemical synthesized in a Russian laboratory to a molecule of medical significance underscores the complex interplay between scientific discovery, regulatory landscapes, and therapeutic innovation.

Today, DMSO continues to be studied for potential new applications, including drug delivery systems, anti-cancer therapies, and as a tool in regenerative medicine. Its rich history reflects the challenges and opportunities inherent in translating chemical compounds from bench to bedside, highlighting the importance of rigorous research and balanced evaluation of risks and benefits.

The Science Behind DMSO: Physical, Chemical, and Pharmacological Properties
Physical Properties

Dimethyl sulfoxide (DMSO) is a highly polar, aprotic solvent known for its exceptional ability to dissolve a wide range of substances, including both polar and nonpolar compounds. It is a colorless, odorless liquid at room temperature, with a molecular weight of 78.13 g/mol. Key physical properties include:

- **Boiling Point**: Approximately 189°C (372°F), indicating its thermal stability.

- **Melting Point**: Around 18.5°C (65°F), which means it solidifies slightly below room temperature.

- **Density**: About 1.1 g/cm³, slightly denser than water.

- **Viscosity**: Low viscosity allows it to penetrate biological membranes efficiently.

- **Hygroscopic Nature**: DMSO is hygroscopic, meaning it readily absorbs moisture from the environment.

Its high dielectric constant (≈47 at 20°C) reflects its ability to stabilize charged species in solution, enhancing its solvent capabilities.

Chemical Properties

Chemically, DMSO is characterized by the presence of a sulfur atom bonded to two methyl groups and double-bonded to an oxygen atom, giving it the formula $(CH_3)_2SO$. This structure imparts several notable chemical properties:

- **Polarity**: The sulfur-oxygen double bond is highly polar, contributing to DMSO's solvent power.

- **Stability**: It is chemically stable under normal conditions but can oxidize to dimethyl sulfone ($DMSO_2$) or reduce to dimethyl sulfide (DMS) under specific conditions.

- **Reactivity**: DMSO is relatively inert but can participate in oxidation-reduction reactions and act as a nucleophile in organic synthesis.

- **Solvent Abilities**: It dissolves many organic and inorganic compounds, including polymers, peptides, and various pharmaceuticals, due to its amphiphilic nature.

Pharmacological Properties

DMSO exhibits a range of pharmacological activities that have been the focus of medical research:

- **Anti-Inflammatory Effects**: It inhibits the formation of inflammatory mediators like prostaglandins and cytokines, reducing inflammation and associated pain.

- **Analgesic Properties**: DMSO can alleviate pain by modulating peripheral nerve conduction and decreasing the release of substance P, a neuropeptide associated with pain signaling.

- **Antioxidant Activity**: Acts as a free radical scavenger, protecting cells from oxidative damage by neutralizing reactive oxygen species (ROS).

- **Membrane Penetration**: Enhances the permeability of biological membranes, facilitating the transdermal delivery of drugs and other therapeutic agents.

- **Cryoprotectant**: Prevents the formation of ice crystals in cells during freezing, making it valuable in cryopreservation of tissues and stem cells.

- **Antimicrobial Action**: Exhibits bacteriostatic and fungistatic properties, inhibiting the growth of certain bacteria and fungi.

- **Radioprotective Effects**: Provides protection against ionizing radiation by scavenging free radicals generated during radiation exposure.

Mechanisms of Action

The therapeutic effects of DMSO are attributed to several mechanisms:

- **Cell Membrane Interaction**: DMSO interacts with lipid bilayers, increasing membrane fluidity and permeability without causing permanent damage. This allows for enhanced transport of molecules across cell membranes.

- **Protein Modulation**: It can influence protein folding and function, affecting enzymes and receptor activities involved in inflammation and pain pathways.

- **Gene Expression**: Alters the expression of certain genes related to inflammation, apoptosis, and cell survival, though the exact pathways are still under investigation.

- **Neurotransmission**: Modulates neural signaling by affecting ion channels and neurotransmitter release, contributing to its analgesic effects.

Pharmacokinetics

Understanding how DMSO is absorbed, distributed, metabolized, and excreted is crucial for its safe use:

- **Absorption**: Rapidly absorbed through the skin, gastrointestinal tract, and mucous membranes due to its low molecular weight and polarity.

- **Distribution**: Widely distributed throughout body tissues, including the central nervous system, owing to its ability to cross the blood-brain barrier.

- **Metabolism**: Primarily metabolized in the liver to dimethyl sulfone ($DMSO_2$), which is excreted in the urine. A smaller fraction is reduced to dimethyl sulfide (DMS), responsible for the characteristic garlic-like odor on the breath and skin.

- **Excretion**: Eliminated via renal excretion, with minor amounts exhaled through the lungs or secreted through sweat glands.

8

Safety Profile and Toxicology

While DMSO is generally considered safe at appropriate concentrations, its potent biological activity necessitates caution:

- **Cytotoxicity**: At high concentrations, DMSO can be cytotoxic, leading to cell lysis and apoptosis.

- **Dermal Reactions**: May cause skin irritation, redness, or dermatitis upon topical application, especially if not properly diluted.

- **Systemic Effects**: Overexposure can lead to headaches, dizziness, nausea, and other systemic symptoms.

- **Drug Interactions**: Due to its carrier properties, DMSO can enhance the absorption of other substances, including toxins, which underscores the importance of ensuring that the skin is clean and free of contaminants before application.

Clinical Implications

The unique combination of physical and chemical properties makes DMSO a versatile agent in medical applications:

- **Drug Delivery Systems**: Its ability to enhance the permeability of biological membranes is utilized in transdermal drug formulations.

- **Anti-Inflammatory Therapies**: Effective in reducing inflammation in conditions like arthritis, bursitis, and tendonitis.

- **Pain Management**: Used for its analgesic properties in musculoskeletal injuries and neuropathic pain.

- **Cryomedicine**: Essential in the preservation of organs, tissues, and cells for transplantation and research.

Ongoing Research

Current scientific investigations are exploring:

- **Cancer Treatment**: Evaluating DMSO's potential to enhance the efficacy of chemotherapeutic agents and its role in apoptosis of cancer cells.

- **Neuroprotection**: Studying its effects in neurodegenerative diseases due to its antioxidant properties and ability to cross the blood-brain barrier.

- **Anti-Microbial Applications**: Assessing its efficacy against resistant bacterial and fungal strains.

Legal Status and FDA Regulations

Overview of Regulatory Status

Dimethyl sulfoxide (DMSO) occupies a unique position in the regulatory landscape of pharmaceuticals and medical treatments. In the United States, the Food and Drug Administration (FDA) has approved DMSO for a very limited set of medical applications, despite its extensive use in research and alternative medicine practices globally.

FDA Approval for Interstitial Cystitis

As of the current regulatory framework, DMSO is officially approved by the FDA for the treatment of interstitial cystitis, a chronic inflammatory condition of the bladder. Marketed under the brand name **Rimso-50**, it is administered intravesically, meaning it is directly instilled into the bladder. The approval came after clinical trials demonstrated its efficacy in alleviating bladder pain and discomfort associated with this condition.

Historical Context of FDA Evaluation

The journey toward FDA approval for other potential uses of DMSO has been fraught with challenges:

- **Initial Interest in the 1960s**: Following promising early research highlighting DMSO's anti-inflammatory and analgesic properties, there was considerable enthusiasm for its medical potential. Preliminary clinical trials explored its use for conditions like musculoskeletal injuries and arthritis.

- **Safety Concerns**: Reports emerged of adverse effects, particularly ocular toxicity observed in animal studies. Specifically, changes in the refractive index of the eye lens in canine models raised red flags about potential vision impairment in humans.

- **Regulatory Hesitation**: Due to these safety concerns, the FDA imposed a temporary moratorium on clinical trials involving DMSO in the mid-1960s. The agency required more comprehensive studies to assess the risks versus benefits.

- **Re-evaluation and Limited Approval**: Subsequent research addressed some safety issues, leading to the approval of DMSO for interstitial cystitis in 1978. However, the FDA remained cautious about expanding its approved uses without robust clinical evidence demonstrating safety and efficacy.

Current Regulatory Limitations

- **Off-Label Use**: While physicians may legally prescribe DMSO off-label for other conditions, such practices are based on clinical judgment rather than FDA approval. The lack of official endorsement means that insurance companies often do not cover off-label uses, and patients may assume greater risk.

- **Over-the-Counter Sales**: DMSO is available in various forms over the counter, typically marketed as a solvent or for veterinary use. Products sold for non-medical purposes are not subject to the same stringent quality controls as pharmaceutical-grade DMSO.

- **Quality and Purity Concerns**: The FDA does not regulate DMSO sold as a dietary supplement or industrial solvent. This lack of oversight can result in variability in purity and concentration, posing potential risks to consumers who use these products for medicinal purposes.

International Regulatory Perspectives

- **Canada and Europe**: Regulatory agencies in other countries have taken a more permissive stance on DMSO. In Canada and several European nations, DMSO is approved for a broader range of medical applications, including as a topical analgesic and anti-inflammatory agent.

- **Global Clinical Trials**: International research continues to explore new therapeutic uses for DMSO, contributing to a growing body of evidence that may influence future regulatory decisions.

FDA Guidelines and Requirements

- **Clinical Trial Requirements**: For any new indication, DMSO must undergo rigorous Phase I-III clinical trials to establish safety and efficacy per FDA guidelines. This process involves:

  - **Phase I**: Assessing safety and dosage in a small group of healthy volunteers.

  - **Phase II**: Evaluating efficacy and side effects in a larger patient group.

  - **Phase III**: Confirming effectiveness, monitoring adverse reactions, and comparing it to commonly used treatments.

- **Good Manufacturing Practices (GMP)**: Pharmaceutical-grade DMSO must be produced following GMP to ensure consistency, purity, and quality.

- **Adverse Event Reporting**: Manufacturers and healthcare providers are required to report any adverse events associated with DMSO use to the FDA's MedWatch program, aiding in post-market surveillance.

Legal Implications for Practitioners and Consumers

- **Healthcare Providers**: Physicians prescribing DMSO off-label must do so with informed consent, discussing potential risks and the lack of FDA approval for specific uses.

- **Consumers**: Individuals using over-the-counter DMSO for self-treatment assume personal responsibility. Without regulatory oversight, they risk exposure to impure products and lack professional guidance on safe usage.

- **Importation of DMSO**: Importing DMSO for personal use may be subject to regulatory scrutiny. The FDA may detain products that do not comply with its regulations.

Chapter 1: Understanding DMSO

How DMSO Works in the Body

Dimethyl sulfoxide (DMSO) exerts its effects in the human body through a combination of unique biochemical interactions and physiological mechanisms. Its multifaceted actions are a result of its ability to interact with biological molecules, influence cellular processes, and modulate physiological responses.

Membrane Interaction and Permeability Enhancement

One of the primary ways DMSO functions is by integrating into biological membranes, altering their physicochemical properties. DMSO interacts with the lipid bilayer of cell membranes, affecting membrane fluidity and permeability without causing significant structural disruption. This interaction occurs due to DMSO's amphiphilic nature, allowing it to associate with both hydrophilic head groups and hydrophobic tail regions of membrane lipids.

- **Mechanism**: DMSO molecules insert themselves between lipid molecules in the membrane, causing expansion and increased disorder within the lipid bilayer. This results in enhanced permeability, allowing for easier passage of ions and small molecules across the membrane.

- **Implications**: The increased permeability facilitates the translocation of therapeutic agents, nutrients, and metabolites into and out of cells, enhancing their bioavailability and efficacy.

Modulation of Signal Transduction Pathways

DMSO influences various intracellular signaling pathways, which can alter cellular responses:

- **Inflammation Pathways**: DMSO inhibits the activation of nuclear factor-kappa B (NF-κB), a transcription factor that regulates the expression of pro-inflammatory cytokines. By suppressing NF-κB activity, DMSO reduces the production of inflammatory mediators such as tumor necrosis factor-alpha (TNF-α) and interleukins.

- **Apoptosis Regulation**: It can induce differentiation and apoptosis in certain cell types by affecting signaling pathways like the mitogen-activated protein kinase (MAPK) pathway.

Antioxidant Activity and Free Radical Scavenging

DMSO acts as a potent scavenger of reactive oxygen species (ROS) and free radicals:

- **Mechanism**: It donates electrons to unstable free radicals, neutralizing them and preventing oxidative damage to cellular components like DNA, proteins, and lipids.

- **Result**: This antioxidant property contributes to cellular protection against oxidative stress, which is implicated in various pathological conditions including inflammation, aging, and cancer.

Interaction with Water Molecules

DMSO's ability to form hydrogen bonds with water molecules affects the hydration shell around proteins and nucleic acids:

- **Protein Folding**: By altering the solvation dynamics, DMSO can influence protein folding and stability, potentially affecting enzyme activities and receptor functions.

- **Nucleic Acid Interactions**: DMSO can intercalate between nucleic acid bases, affecting DNA and RNA stability and transcriptional processes.

Modulation of Immune Responses

DMSO has immunomodulatory effects that impact both innate and adaptive immune systems:

- **Leukocyte Activity**: It inhibits the migration of neutrophils and macrophages to sites of inflammation, reducing tissue damage caused by excessive immune cell infiltration.

- **Cytokine Production**: By modulating cytokine release, DMSO can attenuate hyperactive immune responses, which is beneficial in autoimmune conditions.

Neurotransmission and Pain Perception

DMSO affects neural activity and pain signaling:

- **Ion Channel Modulation**: It influences the function of ion channels, including sodium and calcium channels, which play a role in nerve impulse transmission.

- **Substance P Inhibition**: DMSO reduces the release of substance P, a neuropeptide associated with pain perception, thereby exerting analgesic effects.

Enhancement of Drug Efficacy

As a carrier molecule, DMSO enhances the absorption and efficacy of co-administered drugs:

- **Synergistic Effects**: By increasing the permeability of biological membranes, DMSO allows higher concentrations of drugs to reach target tissues.

- **Pharmacokinetics Alteration**: It can modify the distribution and elimination of drugs, potentially enhancing therapeutic outcomes while necessitating careful dose management.

Cryoprotective Mechanisms

In cryopreservation, DMSO protects cells and tissues from freezing-induced damage:

- **Prevention of Ice Crystal Formation**: DMSO reduces ice nucleation and growth within cells, preventing mechanical damage to cellular structures.

- **Osmotic Balance Maintenance**: It helps in balancing osmotic pressures during the freezing and thawing processes, ensuring cell viability.

Effects on Gene Expression

DMSO can influence gene expression patterns:

- **Epigenetic Modifications**: It affects DNA methylation and histone acetylation status, potentially altering the transcriptional activity of certain genes.

- **Stem Cell Differentiation**: DMSO is used to induce differentiation in stem cell research, guiding cells toward specific lineages by modulating gene expression.

Impact on Enzymatic Activities

By interacting with enzymes, DMSO can modulate metabolic processes:

- **Enzyme Inhibition or Activation**: It may inhibit or enhance the activity of enzymes involved in metabolism, detoxification, and biosynthesis pathways.

- **Metabolic Regulation**: These effects can influence cellular metabolism, impacting energy production and utilization.

Anti-Microbial Actions

DMSO exhibits bacteriostatic and fungistatic properties:

- **Cell Wall Penetration**: It disrupts microbial cell membranes, increasing permeability and leading to loss of vital intracellular components.

- **Synergism with Antimicrobials**: DMSO enhances the effectiveness of antimicrobial agents by facilitating their entry into microbial cells.

Radioprotective Effects

In the context of radiation exposure:

- **Free Radical Neutralization**: DMSO scavenges radiation-induced free radicals, reducing cellular and DNA damage.

- **Protection of Hematopoietic Systems**: It may safeguard bone marrow cells from radiation-induced apoptosis, aiding in the preservation of immune function.

Therapeutic Implications

The diverse mechanisms by which DMSO operates translate into various therapeutic benefits:

- **Anti-Inflammatory Therapy**: By mitigating inflammatory pathways, DMSO serves as an effective agent in conditions characterized by excessive inflammation.

- **Pain Management**: Its analgesic properties offer relief in chronic pain syndromes without the side effects associated with opioid medications.

- **Drug Delivery Enhancement**: DMSO's carrier ability improves the bioavailability of drugs, potentially allowing for lower dosages and reduced side effects.

- **Cell Preservation and Regeneration**: In regenerative medicine, DMSO aids in the preservation of cells and may support tissue repair mechanisms.

Safety Considerations in Physiological Interactions

Understanding how DMSO works in the body is crucial for its safe application:

- **Concentration-Dependent Effects**: The biological activities of DMSO are highly dependent on concentration, with higher levels potentially causing cytotoxicity.

- **Systemic Distribution**: Its ability to cross biological barriers necessitates caution to prevent unintended systemic effects.

- **Interaction with Other Substances**: Due to its solvent properties, DMSO can carry impurities or toxins into the body if not used with pure substances and under sterile conditions.

Benefits and Therapeutic Uses

Dimethyl sulfoxide (DMSO) has garnered significant attention in the medical community due to its diverse pharmacological properties and potential therapeutic applications. This section delves into the scientifically recognized benefits and therapeutic uses of DMSO, emphasizing evidence-based findings while acknowledging areas where further research is warranted.

Approved Medical Applications

Interstitial Cystitis (Bladder Pain Syndrome)

- **Description**: Interstitial cystitis is a chronic condition characterized by bladder pressure, bladder pain, and sometimes pelvic pain, ranging from mild discomfort to severe pain.

- **DMSO's Role**: DMSO is the only FDA-approved intravesical treatment for interstitial cystitis. Administered directly into the bladder via catheter, it serves as a therapeutic agent to alleviate symptoms.

- **Mechanism of Action**:

    o **Anti-Inflammatory Effects**: DMSO reduces inflammation of the bladder wall by inhibiting the release of pro-inflammatory cytokines.

    o **Analgesic Properties**: It diminishes pain signals by modulating nerve conduction.

    o **Muscle Relaxation**: DMSO relaxes bladder muscles, reducing urinary urgency and frequency.

- **Clinical Evidence**: Multiple studies have demonstrated that DMSO instillation leads to symptomatic relief in a significant proportion of patients with interstitial cystitis.

Investigational and Potential Therapeutic Uses

While DMSO is officially approved for interstitial cystitis, its pharmacological properties suggest potential benefits for a variety of other conditions. These uses are considered investigational and should be approached with careful consideration.

Musculoskeletal Disorders

- **Osteoarthritis and Rheumatoid Arthritis**:
  - **Benefits**: Topical application of DMSO may reduce joint pain and swelling due to its anti-inflammatory and analgesic effects.
  - **Evidence**: Some clinical trials and patient reports indicate symptomatic improvement; however, large-scale, randomized controlled trials are lacking.

- **Tendinitis and Bursitis**:
  - **Benefits**: DMSO may alleviate inflammation of tendons and bursae when applied topically.
  - **Evidence**: Limited studies suggest potential benefits, but more rigorous research is needed to confirm efficacy.

Dermatological Conditions

- **Scleroderma**:
  - **Benefits**: DMSO may soften hardened skin and improve mobility in affected areas.
  - **Evidence**: Early studies showed promise, but subsequent research provided mixed results, necessitating further investigation.

- **Herpes Zoster (Shingles)**:
  - **Benefits**: When combined with antiviral medications, DMSO may enhance drug penetration and reduce pain and healing time.
  - **Evidence**: Preliminary studies are encouraging but not definitive.

Pain Management

- **Neuropathic Pain**:
  - **Benefits**: DMSO's ability to modulate nerve function suggests potential in treating neuropathic pain conditions.
  - **Evidence**: Animal models demonstrate analgesic effects; human studies are minimal and inconclusive.

Inflammatory Conditions

- **Soft Tissue Injuries**:
  - **Benefits**: Application of DMSO may reduce inflammation and expedite healing in sprains, strains, and bruises.
  - **Evidence**: Anecdotal reports and small studies support its use, but comprehensive clinical data are insufficient.

Cryopreservation

- **Cell and Tissue Preservation**:
  - **Benefits**: DMSO is widely used as a cryoprotectant to preserve cells, tissues, and organs at low temperatures.
  - **Mechanism**: It prevents ice crystal formation, protecting cellular integrity during freezing and thawing processes.
  - **Evidence**: Its efficacy is well-established in laboratory and clinical settings, particularly in stem cell transplantation.

Potential Antioxidant Effects

- **Oxidative Stress-Related Disorders**:

14

- o **Benefits**: DMSO may protect cells from oxidative damage by scavenging free radicals.

- o **Evidence**: Laboratory studies confirm antioxidant properties; clinical implications remain speculative.

Central Nervous System Injuries

- **Traumatic Brain Injury and Spinal Cord Injury**:

  - o **Benefits**: DMSO may reduce edema and secondary injury mechanisms when administered promptly after trauma.

  - o **Evidence**: Results from animal studies are promising; human clinical trials are limited and have not led to standard treatment protocols.

Gastrointestinal Disorders

- **Ulcerative Colitis and Proctitis**:

  - o **Benefits**: Rectal administration of DMSO might reduce inflammation in the lower gastrointestinal tract.

  - o **Evidence**: Small-scale studies indicate potential benefits, but larger, controlled trials are necessary.

Antimicrobial Properties

- **Infections**:

  - o **Benefits**: DMSO exhibits bacteriostatic and fungistatic activities, potentially enhancing the effectiveness of antimicrobial agents.

  - o **Evidence**: In vitro studies demonstrate antimicrobial effects; clinical relevance has yet to be established.

Enhancing Drug Delivery

- **Transdermal Drug Administration**:

  - o **Benefits**: DMSO increases skin permeability, potentially improving the absorption of co-administered topical medications.

  - o **Applications**: Used experimentally to deliver steroids, nonsteroidal anti-inflammatory drugs (NSAIDs), and other agents.

  - o **Evidence**: Some studies show enhanced drug efficacy; safety and optimal formulations require further research.

Anti-Cancer Research

- **Cancer Therapy Adjunct**:

  - o **Benefits**: DMSO may induce differentiation in certain malignant cells and enhance the effectiveness of chemotherapy agents.

  - o **Evidence**: Laboratory studies reveal potential anti-cancer mechanisms; clinical applications are unproven and experimental.

Veterinary Medicine Applications

- **Equine and Canine Treatments**:

  - o **Benefits**: DMSO is utilized to treat inflammation, swelling, and certain neurological conditions in animals.

  - o **Evidence**: Widely accepted in veterinary practice, with documented benefits in reducing cerebral edema and treating laminitis in horses.

Safety Profile and Considerations

While exploring the therapeutic uses of DMSO, it is crucial to consider its safety profile:

- **Adverse Effects**:

    o **Dermal Reactions**: Skin irritation, redness, and dermatitis may occur with topical use.

    o **Systemic Effects**: Headaches, dizziness, and gastrointestinal disturbances have been reported with higher doses.

    o **Odor**: A characteristic garlic-like odor on the breath and skin results from dimethyl sulfide, a metabolite of DMSO.

- **Drug Interactions**: DMSO's solvent properties may alter the absorption and efficacy of other medications.

- **Purity and Quality**: Pharmaceutical-grade DMSO should be used to minimize the risk of contaminants.

Current Research and Future Directions

- **Clinical Trials**: Ongoing studies aim to better understand DMSO's efficacy and safety in various therapeutic contexts.

- **Novel Applications**: Research into DMSO derivatives and formulations seeks to enhance its beneficial properties while reducing adverse effects.

- **Regulatory Evaluation**: Accumulating scientific evidence may inform future regulatory decisions regarding additional approved uses.

Common Misconceptions and Myths

Despite extensive research and documented uses, dimethyl sulfoxide (DMSO) is surrounded by several misconceptions and myths that can lead to misunderstanding or misuse. This section aims to clarify common misconceptions by providing evidence-based explanations.

Misconception 1: DMSO Is a Miracle Cure for All Ailments

Clarification: While DMSO has demonstrated therapeutic potential in various conditions due to its anti-inflammatory and analgesic properties, it is not a panacea. Its efficacy is primarily established for specific applications, such as the treatment of interstitial cystitis. Claims that DMSO can cure a wide range of diseases, including cancer or neurodegenerative disorders, are not supported by sufficient clinical evidence. Overstating its capabilities can lead individuals to forego proven treatments in favor of unverified uses.

Misconception 2: DMSO Is Completely Safe Without Any Side Effects

Clarification: No therapeutic agent is entirely free of side effects, and DMSO is no exception. Common side effects include skin irritation, redness, and a garlic-like odor on the breath and skin due to its metabolism to dimethyl sulfide. High concentrations or improper use can lead to more severe reactions, such as headaches, dizziness, or allergic responses. It is essential to use DMSO under appropriate guidance and to adhere to recommended concentrations to minimize risks.

Misconception 3: All Grades of DMSO Are Suitable for Medical Use

Clarification: DMSO is available in various grades, including industrial-grade and pharmaceutical-grade. Industrial-grade DMSO may contain impurities and contaminants unsuitable for medical applications. Only pharmaceutical-grade DMSO, which meets strict purity standards, should be used for therapeutic purposes. Utilizing lower-grade products can introduce harmful substances into the body, leading to adverse effects.

Misconception 4: DMSO Can Be Used Without Medical Supervision

Clarification: Self-administering DMSO without professional guidance can be hazardous. Due to its potent solvent properties and ability to enhance the absorption of other substances, incorrect usage can result in unintended systemic exposure to toxins or medications. Medical supervision ensures proper dosing, application methods, and monitoring for potential interactions or side effects.

Misconception 5: Topical DMSO Does Not Require Dilution

Clarification: Applying undiluted DMSO (100% concentration) to the skin can increase the risk of irritation, burning sensations, and dermatitis. Appropriate dilution is crucial and varies depending on the intended use. For most topical applications, concentrations between 50% and 70% are commonly recommended. Diluting DMSO with sterile water or other compatible solvents helps reduce adverse skin reactions while maintaining therapeutic effectiveness.

Misconception 6: DMSO Can Transport Any Substance Through the Skin Safely

Clarification: While DMSO enhances the permeability of the skin, it does not discriminate between beneficial and harmful substances. It can facilitate the transdermal absorption of contaminants, pathogens, or chemicals present on the skin's surface. Therefore, it is imperative to ensure the skin is thoroughly cleansed before application and to avoid combining DMSO with substances not intended for systemic absorption.

Misconception 7: There Is Extensive Clinical Evidence Supporting All Uses of DMSO

Clarification: Although DMSO has been studied for various potential applications, robust clinical evidence is limited to certain conditions. Many purported benefits are based on preliminary studies, anecdotal reports, or in vitro research. High-quality, large-scale clinical trials are lacking for many off-label uses. Relying on unverified claims can lead to ineffective treatment or delay in receiving appropriate medical care.

Misconception 8: DMSO Does Not Interact with Other Medications

Clarification: DMSO's ability to alter membrane permeability can affect the absorption and efficacy of concomitant medications. It may potentiate or diminish the effects of certain drugs, leading to unforeseen therapeutic outcomes or side effects. It is crucial to discuss the use of DMSO with a healthcare provider, especially when taking other medications, to assess potential interactions.

Misconception 9: Oral Consumption of DMSO Is Universally Safe and Effective

Clarification: Oral administration of DMSO is not well-established and may pose risks such as gastrointestinal irritation or systemic toxicity. The safety profile for oral consumption has not been thoroughly evaluated in clinical settings. Until more definitive research is available, oral use of DMSO should be approached with caution and under professional supervision.

Misconception 10: DMSO Use Is Suppressed by the Medical Community or Pharmaceutical Industry

Clarification: Conspiracy theories suggesting that DMSO is intentionally suppressed lack credible evidence. Regulatory agencies like the FDA require rigorous scientific validation to approve substances for medical use. DMSO's approval for specific applications, such as interstitial cystitis, reflects the current level of evidence supporting its safety and efficacy. Ongoing research continues to explore additional therapeutic uses, and regulatory decisions are based on emerging scientific data.

Misconception 11: DMSO Does Not Cause Any Odor

Clarification: A common side effect of DMSO use is the development of a garlic-like odor on the breath and skin. This occurs because DMSO is metabolized into dimethyl sulfide, a compound with a strong odor. This side effect is harmless but can be socially inconvenient. Users should be aware of this possibility and understand that it is a normal consequence of DMSO metabolism.

Misconception 12: Children and Pregnant Women Can Use DMSO Without Concern

Clarification: The safety of DMSO in children and during pregnancy or breastfeeding has not been adequately studied. Due to the lack of data on its effects on fetal development or in pediatric populations, DMSO use in these groups should be avoided unless specifically recommended and supervised by a qualified healthcare professional.

Precautions and Safety Measures

The therapeutic use of dimethyl sulfoxide (DMSO) requires careful consideration of various safety measures to minimize potential risks and adverse effects. This section outlines the essential precautions and guidelines for the safe handling and application of DMSO, based on current scientific understanding.

Selection of Appropriate DMSO Grade

- **Pharmaceutical-Grade DMSO**: Always use pharmaceutical-grade DMSO for medical applications. This grade meets stringent purity standards, reducing the risk of contaminants that may cause adverse reactions.

- **Avoid Industrial-Grade DMSO**: Industrial-grade DMSO may contain impurities and should not be used for therapeutic purposes due to potential toxicity.

Dilution and Concentration Guidelines

- **Proper Dilution**: DMSO should be diluted to appropriate concentrations before use. Common concentrations for topical applications range from 25% to 70%, depending on the condition being treated.

- **Use of Sterile Diluents**: Dilute DMSO with sterile, distilled water or saline to prevent contamination. Avoid tap water or non-sterile liquids that may introduce pathogens or impurities.

- **Concentration Selection**: Choose the concentration based on therapeutic needs and tolerance levels. Higher concentrations may increase the risk of skin irritation and other adverse effects.

Skin Preparation and Application

- **Thorough Cleaning of Application Site**: Clean the skin thoroughly with mild soap and water before applying DMSO. This step removes dirt, oils, and potential contaminants that could be absorbed transdermally.

- **Avoid Contaminants**: Do not apply lotions, creams, or other topical products before or immediately after DMSO application, as DMSO may facilitate their systemic absorption.

- **Protective Gloves**: Wear disposable gloves when handling DMSO to prevent unintended absorption through the hands and to maintain hygiene.

- **Test for Sensitivity**: Conduct a patch test by applying a small amount of diluted DMSO to a small skin area to check for allergic reactions or sensitivity before widespread use.

Application Techniques

- **Use Clean Applicators**: Apply DMSO using sterile cotton swabs, gauze pads, or glass applicators. Avoid materials that may react with DMSO, such as certain plastics or metals.

- **Avoid Open Wounds**: Do not apply DMSO to open wounds, broken skin, or mucous membranes unless under medical supervision, as it may cause irritation or systemic absorption of contaminants.

- **Dosage Control**: Adhere to recommended dosage guidelines. Overapplication may increase the risk of adverse effects without providing additional therapeutic benefits.

Managing Adverse Effects

- **Skin Irritation**: Monitor for signs of skin irritation, such as redness, itching, or burning sensations. If irritation occurs, discontinue use or reduce the concentration.

- **Garlic-like Odor**: Be aware that DMSO metabolism can cause a temporary garlic-like odor on the breath and skin. This is a normal effect and typically subsides after discontinuation.

- **Systemic Reactions**: Watch for systemic symptoms like headaches, dizziness, or gastrointestinal discomfort. Seek medical advice if such symptoms develop.

Drug Interactions and Concomitant Medications

- **Consult Healthcare Professionals**: Inform healthcare providers about all medications and supplements being taken to assess potential interactions.

- **Enhanced Absorption**: Recognize that DMSO can enhance the absorption of other drugs, potentially altering their efficacy or increasing the risk of side effects.

- **Avoid Alcohol and Certain Drugs**: Limit alcohol consumption and be cautious with medications that have a narrow therapeutic index or are known to interact with DMSO.

18

Special Populations

- **Pregnancy and Breastfeeding**: The safety of DMSO during pregnancy and lactation has not been established. Avoid use unless prescribed and supervised by a qualified healthcare professional.

- **Children**: Use in pediatric populations should be under strict medical supervision, with careful consideration of appropriate dosing and potential risks.

- **Elderly Patients**: Older adults may have increased sensitivity and should use lower concentrations with monitoring for adverse effects.

Storage and Handling

- **Proper Storage**: Store DMSO in a cool, dry place away from direct sunlight to maintain its stability. Keep the container tightly closed to prevent contamination.

- **Container Materials**: Use storage containers made of compatible materials, such as glass or certain types of plastic (e.g., high-density polyethylene), to prevent reactions with the solvent.

- **Keep Out of Reach of Children**: Ensure that DMSO is stored securely to prevent accidental ingestion or misuse by children or pets.

Environmental Considerations

- **Disposal**: Dispose of unused DMSO and contaminated materials in accordance with local regulations. Avoid pouring large quantities down the drain or into the environment.

- **Spill Management**: In case of spills, clean the area with absorbent materials and ventilate the space to dissipate vapors.

Medical Supervision and Legal Compliance

- **Professional Guidance**: Use DMSO under the guidance of a qualified healthcare professional, especially for internal use or treating serious conditions.

- **Regulatory Awareness**: Be aware of the legal status of DMSO in your region and comply with regulations regarding its purchase and therapeutic use.

Allergic Reactions and Contraindications

- **Hypersensitivity**: Individuals with known allergies to DMSO should not use it. Signs of allergic reactions include rash, hives, difficulty breathing, or swelling.

- **Contraindicated Conditions**: Use caution or avoid DMSO in conditions such as severe liver or kidney impairment, as metabolism and excretion may be affected.

Monitoring and Follow-Up

- **Regular Assessment**: Monitor the treated condition for improvement or signs of adverse reactions. Adjust usage accordingly in consultation with a healthcare provider.

- **Laboratory Tests**: In cases of prolonged use or higher dosages, periodic laboratory tests may be recommended to assess organ function and overall health.

Education and Informed Use

- **Stay Informed**: Keep updated with the latest research and recommendations regarding DMSO use.

- **Informed Consent**: Understand the potential benefits and risks before initiating treatment, making informed decisions based on current scientific evidence.

Chapter 2: Getting Started with DMSO

Types and Grades of DMSO

Dimethyl sulfoxide (DMSO) is available in various types and grades, each distinguished by its purity level, intended use, and manufacturing standards. Selecting the appropriate grade of DMSO is critical for ensuring safety and efficacy, particularly when used for medical or therapeutic purposes.

Purity Grades

DMSO is classified into different purity grades based on the level of contaminants and the rigorousness of purification processes:

Industrial Grade (Technical Grade)

- **Purity Level**: Typically ranges from 90% to 98%.

- **Intended Use**: Designed for industrial applications such as solvent extraction, chemical synthesis, and manufacturing processes.

- **Characteristics**:

    o   Contains higher levels of impurities, including trace metals and organic contaminants.

    o   Not subjected to stringent purification protocols.

- **Risks**:

    o   Unsuitable for medical or therapeutic use due to potential toxicity from contaminants.

    o   Increased risk of adverse reactions if applied to biological systems.

Pharmaceutical Grade (Medical Grade)

- **Purity Level**: Generally exceeds 99.5% purity.

- **Intended Use**: Approved for medical applications, including topical treatments, drug formulations, and clinical research.

- **Characteristics**:

    o   Undergoes extensive purification processes to eliminate impurities.

    o   Meets strict quality standards set by pharmacopeias such as the United States Pharmacopeia (USP) or European Pharmacopoeia (EP).

- **Benefits**:

    o   Reduced risk of adverse reactions due to high purity.

    o   Suitable for human use under professional supervision.

Reagent Grade (Analytical Grade)

- **Purity Level**: Exceeds 99.9% purity.

- **Intended Use**: Employed in laboratory settings for analytical procedures, spectroscopy, and high-precision experiments.

- **Characteristics**:

    o   Highest level of purity with minimal impurities.

    o   Ideal for sensitive applications requiring exacting standards.

- **Considerations**:

    o   While extremely pure, it may be more costly.

- Can be used therapeutically if it meets pharmaceutical standards.

Physical Forms

DMSO is available in several physical forms, tailored to specific applications:

Liquid Form

- **Description**: A clear, colorless liquid at room temperature.
- **Applications**:
  - Commonly used for dilution to prepare solutions of varying concentrations.
  - Suitable for both topical application and as a solvent in pharmaceutical formulations.
- **Handling**:
  - Hygroscopic nature necessitates storage in airtight containers.
  - Should be kept away from light and moisture to maintain stability.

Gel Formulations

- **Description**: DMSO combined with gelling agents to create a semi-solid consistency.
- **Applications**:
  - Facilitates easy topical application without running or dripping.
  - Used for localized treatment of pain, inflammation, and skin conditions.
- **Considerations**:
  - Check for additional ingredients that may affect absorption or cause allergic reactions.

Creams and Ointments

- **Description**: Emulsions containing DMSO, water, and lipid components.
- **Applications**:
  - Provide moisturization along with therapeutic effects.
  - Suitable for dermatological applications requiring gradual absorption.
- **Formulation Factors**:
  - Emulsion stability and compatibility with other active ingredients are crucial.
  - Preservatives may be added to extend shelf life.

Concentration Variants

DMSO products come in various concentrations, indicating the percentage of DMSO in the solution:

99% to 100% Concentration

- **Use**: Primarily as a stock solution for dilution to desired concentrations.
- **Caution**:
  - Direct application is not recommended due to the high risk of skin irritation and systemic toxicity.
  - Requires accurate dilution before therapeutic use.

70% to 90% Concentration

- **Use**: May be used in certain clinical settings under professional supervision.
- **Applications**:

- Sometimes employed in research or specialized treatments.
- **Risks**:
    - Higher potential for adverse skin reactions.
    - Not typically recommended for general therapeutic use.

25% to 70% Concentration

- **Use**: Commonly used range for topical therapeutic applications.
- **Applications**:
    - Treatment of musculoskeletal pain, inflammation, and skin disorders.
- **Advantages**:
    - Balances efficacy with a lower risk of irritation.
    - Allows for flexibility in dosing based on patient tolerance.

Below 25% Concentration

- **Use**: Suitable for sensitive skin areas or when minimal penetration is required.
- **Applications**:
    - Pediatric use (under medical supervision).
    - Mild conditions requiring gentle intervention.

Specialized Formulations

DMSO is often combined with other substances to enhance its therapeutic properties:

DMSO with Aloe Vera

- **Purpose**: Aloe vera acts as a soothing agent, reducing potential skin irritation from DMSO.
- **Applications**:
    - Topical treatments for skin conditions.
- **Considerations**:
    - Ensure aloe vera is pure and free from additives.

DMSO with Essential Oils

- **Purpose**: Essential oils may provide additional therapeutic effects and mask the odor of DMSO.
- **Applications**:
    - Aromatherapy and topical treatments.
- **Risks**:
    - Potential for allergic reactions.
    - Enhanced systemic absorption of essential oils, which may not be desirable.

DMSO with Pharmaceutical Agents

- **Purpose**: Enhances the transdermal delivery of medications like anti-inflammatories or analgesics.
- **Applications**:
    - Formulated in prescription medications.

- **Regulatory Status**:
    - Such combinations require approval from regulatory bodies.
    - Safety and efficacy must be established through clinical trials.

Veterinary Grades

- **Intended Use**: Formulated specifically for veterinary applications.
- **Characteristics**:
    - May have different purity standards compared to human pharmaceutical grade.
- **Applications**:
    - Used in animals for conditions like joint pain and inflammation.
- **Caution**:
    - Not recommended for human use due to potential differences in purity and additives.

Selection Guidelines for Therapeutic Use

When choosing a DMSO product for medical purposes, consider the following:

Purity Verification

- **Certificates of Analysis (CoA)**:
    - Request CoA from manufacturers to confirm purity levels.
- **Reputable Suppliers**:
    - Purchase from established suppliers who adhere to Good Manufacturing Practices (GMP).

Intended Application

- **Topical Use**:
    - Select appropriate concentration and formulation (e.g., gel, cream).
- **Internal Use**:
    - Only under strict medical supervision, using pharmaceutical-grade DMSO.

Compatibility with Other Substances

- **Additives and Excipients**:
    - Review all ingredients for potential allergens or irritants.
- **Drug Interactions**:
    - Consult healthcare providers about concomitant medications.

Regulatory Compliance

- **Legal Status**:
    - Ensure the product complies with local regulations for medical use.
- **Labeling Standards**:
    - Verify that labeling includes necessary information such as concentration, purity, and usage instructions.

Storage and Handling

- **Container Material**:

o   Store DMSO in glass or compatible plastic containers to prevent reactions.

- **Temperature Control**:

    o   Keep in a cool, dry place away from direct sunlight.

- **Avoid Contamination**:

    o   Use clean equipment when handling to maintain purity.

Pharmaceutical Grade vs. Industrial Grade

Understanding the distinction between pharmaceutical grade and industrial grade dimethyl sulfoxide (DMSO) is essential for ensuring safety and efficacy in therapeutic applications. These two grades differ significantly in terms of purity, manufacturing standards, intended use, and regulatory oversight. Selecting the appropriate grade is crucial to minimize health risks and achieve the desired therapeutic outcomes.

Pharmaceutical Grade DMSO

Purity and Quality Standards

- **High Purity Levels**: Pharmaceutical grade DMSO typically has a purity of ≥99.5%, often reaching up to **99.99%**. This high purity is achieved through rigorous purification processes that remove impurities and contaminants.

- **Regulatory Compliance**: It adheres to strict standards set by pharmacopeias such as the **United States Pharmacopeia (USP), European Pharmacopoeia (EP)**, or **Japanese Pharmacopoeia (JP)**.

- **Good Manufacturing Practices (GMP)**: Produced in facilities that comply with GMP guidelines, ensuring consistent quality, traceability, and adherence to safety protocols.

Quality Control Measures

- **Analytical Testing**: Undergoes extensive testing using techniques like gas chromatography and mass spectrometry to detect impurities, including heavy metals and residual solvents.

- **Certificates of Analysis (CoA)**: Each batch is accompanied by a CoA that details purity levels, impurity profiles, and compliance with regulatory standards.

Intended Use

- **Medical Applications**: Specifically formulated for therapeutic use in humans, including topical treatments, injectable formulations (where approved), and as a carrier solvent in pharmaceuticals.

- **Safety Profile**: The high purity minimizes the risk of adverse reactions related to contaminants, making it suitable for clinical settings.

Packaging and Handling

- **Sterile Packaging**: Often packaged in sterile, medical-grade containers to prevent contamination.

- **Labeling:** Clearly labeled with concentration, purity level, lot number, expiration date, and storage instructions.

Industrial Grade DMSO

Purity and Quality Standards

- **Lower Purity Levels**: Industrial grade DMSO generally has a purity ranging from **90% to 98%**.

- **Presence of Impurities**: May contain higher levels of organic and inorganic impurities, including heavy metals and other chemical residues.

- **Lack of Regulatory Oversight**: Does not comply with pharmacopeial standards and lacks stringent quality control measures.

Quality Control Measures

- **Limited Testing**: Quality assessments focus on parameters relevant to industrial applications, not on purity levels required for medical use.
- **No Certificates of Analysis**: Often lacks detailed documentation of impurity profiles and may not provide CoAs.

Intended Use

- **Industrial Applications**: Designed for use as a solvent in manufacturing processes, chemical synthesis, paint stripping, cleaning agents, and other industrial activities.
- **Not for Human Use**: Not intended or safe for therapeutic use due to potential toxicity from impurities.

Packaging and Handling

- **Non-Sterile Packaging**: Packaged in containers suitable for industrial storage, which may not prevent contamination by environmental factors.
- **Labeling**: Labels may not include detailed information on purity, concentration, or safe handling instructions for medical use.

Risks Associated with Using Industrial Grade DMSO Medically

Health Hazards

- **Toxic Impurities**: Contaminants such as heavy metals (lead, arsenic, mercury) and organic solvents can cause serious health issues, including organ toxicity and carcinogenic effects.
- **Enhanced Absorption of Contaminants**: DMSO's ability to penetrate biological membranes can facilitate the systemic absorption of impurities, increasing the risk of adverse reactions.
- **Unpredictable Reactions**: The presence of unknown contaminants may lead to unexpected pharmacological effects or interfere with normal physiological processes.

Lack of Safety Data

- **No Clinical Testing**: Industrial grade DMSO has not been tested for safety or efficacy in humans.
- **Inconsistent Quality**: Variability between batches can result in inconsistent therapeutic outcomes and increase the potential for harm.

Legal and Ethical Considerations

- **Regulatory Non-Compliance**: Using industrial grade DMSO for medical purposes may violate regulatory laws and guidelines.
- **Professional Liability**: Healthcare providers recommending or administering industrial grade DMSO may face legal repercussions and ethical violations.

Advantages of Using Pharmaceutical Grade DMSO

Safety Assurance

- **Minimized Contaminants**: High purification standards reduce the presence of harmful substances.
- **Predictable Pharmacokinetics**: Consistent purity ensures reliable absorption, distribution, metabolism, and excretion profiles.

Efficacy

- **Therapeutic Consistency**: Purity leads to consistent therapeutic effects, enabling accurate dosing and monitoring.
- **Clinical Validation**: Pharmaceutical grade DMSO is supported by clinical studies and approved for certain medical uses (e.g., treatment of interstitial cystitis).

Regulatory Compliance

- **Legal Use**: Complies with laws and regulations governing pharmaceutical substances.

- **Quality Assurance**: Adherence to GMP and pharmacopeial standards provides confidence in the product's integrity.

Practical Guidelines for Selecting the Appropriate Grade

For Healthcare Providers

- **Prescription Practices**: Prescribe only pharmaceutical grade DMSO for therapeutic applications.

- **Patient Education**: Inform patients about the importance of using the correct grade and the risks associated with industrial grade products.

- **Verification**: Ensure that suppliers provide pharmaceutical grade DMSO with appropriate documentation.

For Consumers

- **Product Labels**: Check labels carefully for indications of pharmaceutical grade and compliance with pharmacopeial standards.

- **Supplier Reputation**: Purchase from reputable pharmacies or medical suppliers known for quality products.

- **Avoid Unverified Sources**: Be cautious of online vendors or retailers selling DMSO without proper labeling or quality assurances.

Purity and Concentrations

Importance of Purity in DMSO

The purity of dimethyl sulfoxide (DMSO) is a critical factor that directly impacts its safety and efficacy in medical applications. High-purity DMSO ensures that the compound is free from contaminants that could cause adverse reactions or interfere with its therapeutic properties. Impurities may include residual solvents, heavy metals, or other organic compounds that can pose significant health risks when introduced into the body.

Quantifying Purity

Purity is typically expressed as a percentage, indicating the proportion of DMSO in the product relative to all other substances present. Pharmaceutical-grade DMSO generally exhibits a purity of **≥99.5%**, often reaching up to **99.99%**. This high level of purity is achieved through rigorous purification processes and stringent quality control measures. Analytical techniques used to assess purity include:

- **Gas Chromatography (GC)**: Separates and quantifies volatile impurities.

- **High-Performance Liquid Chromatography (HPLC)**: Detects non-volatile organic contaminants.

- **Inductively Coupled Plasma Mass Spectrometry (ICP-MS)**: Measures trace levels of heavy metals.

- **Infrared Spectroscopy (IR)**: Identifies functional groups and detects specific impurities.

Potential Impurities and Their Risks

- **Residual Solvents**: Trace amounts of solvents like methanol or acetone used during manufacturing can remain in the final product, leading to toxicity or allergic reactions.

- **Heavy Metals**: Metals such as lead, arsenic, or mercury can cause organ damage, neurological issues, and other severe health problems even at low concentrations.

- **Organic Impurities**: Unreacted starting materials or by-products can interfere with DMSO's therapeutic action and may introduce additional risks.

Regulatory Standards for Purity

Regulatory agencies such as the **United States Pharmacopeia (USP)** and the **European Pharmacopoeia (EP)** set strict standards for the purity of pharmaceutical-grade DMSO. These standards specify acceptable limits for various impurities and mandate comprehensive testing protocols. Compliance with these regulations ensures that the DMSO is suitable for medical use.

Concentrations of DMSO Solutions

In therapeutic applications, DMSO is rarely used in its pure form; instead, it is diluted to specific concentrations appropriate for the intended use. Concentration refers to the amount of DMSO present in a solution relative to the total volume, usually expressed as a percentage (%).

Common Concentrations and Their Applications

- **90%–99% Concentration**: Generally used as stock solutions or in specialized clinical settings under strict medical supervision. High concentrations can cause skin irritation and are not typically applied directly.

- **70%–90% Concentration**: Employed for certain topical applications where deeper penetration is required, such as severe musculoskeletal injuries.

- **50%–70% Concentration**: Commonly used for general topical treatments, including arthritis pain relief and inflammation reduction.

- **25%–50% Concentration**: Suitable for sensitive skin areas or for individuals who may experience irritation at higher concentrations.

- **10%–25% Concentration**: Used for delicate applications, such as facial treatments or in pediatric care under professional guidance.

How to Dilute DMSO Safely

Diluting dimethyl sulfoxide (DMSO) safely is a critical step in preparing it for therapeutic applications. Proper dilution ensures the desired therapeutic concentration is achieved while minimizing the risk of adverse reactions. This section provides a comprehensive guide on how to dilute DMSO safely, emphasizing best practices, necessary equipment, and safety precautions.

Understanding the Importance of Safe Dilution

- **Therapeutic Efficacy**: Accurate dilution is essential to attain the specific concentration required for the intended therapeutic effect.

- **Minimizing Adverse Effects**: Overly concentrated solutions can cause skin irritation, burns, or systemic toxicity.

- **Consistency**: Precise dilution techniques ensure consistent results across different preparations and applications.

Selecting the Appropriate Diluents

Choosing the correct diluent is crucial for maintaining the stability and efficacy of the DMSO solution.

- **Sterile Distilled Water**: Preferred for most topical applications due to its purity and compatibility.

- **Physiological Saline (0.9% Sodium Chloride Solution)**: Ideal for solutions intended for parenteral administration or when isotonicity is necessary.

- **Buffered Solutions**: In certain cases, a buffered diluent may be required to maintain pH stability.

- **Compatibility Considerations**: Ensure the diluent does not react chemically with DMSO or alter its properties.

Equipment and Materials Needed

- **Personal Protective Equipment (PPE)**:
  - Nitrile or latex gloves
  - Safety goggles

- o Lab coat or apron
- **Measuring Instruments**:
  - o Volumetric flasks or graduated cylinders
  - o Pipettes (mechanical or volumetric)
  - o Syringes with precise gradations
- **Mixing Containers**:
  - o Glass beakers or flasks (preferably amber-colored to protect from light)
  - o Containers made of DMSO-compatible plastics like polypropylene
- **Stirring Devices**:
  - o Magnetic stirrer
  - o Glass stirring rods
- **Storage Containers**:
  - o Airtight, amber glass bottles for storing the diluted solution
  - o Containers should be labeled appropriately

Safety Precautions Before Dilution

- **Work Area Preparation**:
  - o Perform dilution in a well-ventilated area to prevent inhalation of vapors.
  - o Use a clean, uncluttered workspace to reduce the risk of contamination.
- **Personal Hygiene**:
  - o Wash hands thoroughly before and after handling DMSO.
  - o Avoid touching the face or skin during the dilution process.
- **Avoid Contamination**:
  - o Ensure all equipment is clean and, if necessary, sterilized.
  - o Use sterile techniques if preparing solutions for applications requiring sterility.

Step-by-Step Dilution Procedure

1. **Calculate the Required Volumes**:
   - o Determine the desired final concentration and volume of the DMSO solution.
   - o Use the dilution formula:

$$V_{DMSO} = \frac{C_{FINAL} \times V_{FINAL}}{C_{STOCK}}$$

   - - V_{DMSO} = Volume of stock DMSO needed
     - C_{FINAL} = Desired final concentration (%)
     - V_{FINAL} = Desired final total volume
     - C_{STOCK} = Concentration of stock DMSO (usually close to 100%)

2. **Measure the Diluents**:
   - o Using a clean graduated cylinder or volumetric flask, measure the required volume of the diluent.

28

- Pour the diluent into the mixing container.

3. **Measure the DMSO**:
    - Carefully measure the calculated volume of stock DMSO using a clean pipette or syringe.
    - DMSO is hygroscopic and can absorb moisture; minimize exposure to air.

4. **Add DMSO to the Diluent**:
    - **Important**: Always add DMSO to the diluent, not the other way around, to better control the exothermic reaction.
    - Add the DMSO slowly while stirring the diluent gently to promote even mixing and dissipate heat.

5. **Mix Thoroughly**:
    - Continue stirring until the solution is homogeneous.
    - Ensure no layering or separation is visible.

6. **Allow the Solution to Reach Room Temperature**:
    - The mixing process may generate heat. Let the solution cool to room temperature before use.

7. **Transfer to Storage Container**:
    - If not using immediately, transfer the solution to a labeled, airtight container.
    - Include information such as concentration, date of preparation, and expiration date.

Handling Exothermic Reactions

- **Awareness of Heat Generation**: Mixing DMSO with water is exothermic and releases heat.
- **Mitigation Strategies**:
    - Add DMSO slowly to the diluent.
    - Use ice baths for larger volumes to control temperature.
    - Avoid rapid mixing or adding large volumes at once.

Storage of Diluted DMSO Solutions

- **Container Selection**:
    - Use amber glass bottles to protect from light-induced degradation.
    - Ensure the container has a tight seal to prevent absorption of moisture or contaminants.
- **Labeling**:
    - Clearly label the container with all relevant information.
- **Storage Conditions**:
    - Store at controlled room temperature unless otherwise specified.
    - Keep away from direct sunlight and sources of heat.
- **Shelf Life**:
    - Diluted solutions may have a limited shelf life; consult stability data or prepare fresh solutions as needed.

Disposal of Excess or Waste DMSO

- **Follow Local Regulations**: Dispose of DMSO waste according to local environmental and safety regulations.

- **Avoid Environmental Contamination**:
    - Do not pour large quantities down the drain.
    - Use designated chemical waste containers.

Special Considerations

- **Avoiding Contamination**:
    - Do not reuse measuring devices or containers without proper cleaning.
    - Use separate equipment for different substances to prevent cross-contamination.
- **Materials Compatibility**:
    - DMSO can dissolve certain plastics and rubbers; verify that all equipment is compatible.
- **Preventing Skin Contact**:
    - DMSO readily penetrates the skin and can carry contaminants into the bloodstream.
    - Wear gloves and avoid skin contact with both the concentrated and diluted solutions.

Addressing Common Issues

- **Cloudiness or Precipitation**:
    - If the solution becomes cloudy or precipitates form, it may indicate incompatibility or contamination.
    - Discard and prepare a fresh solution.
- **pH Adjustments**:
    - DMSO solutions are typically neutral, but if pH adjustment is necessary, use compatible buffering agents.
    - Avoid introducing substances that may react with DMSO.

Example Dilution Calculation

Objective: Prepare 50 mL of a 30% DMSO solution from pure DMSO (assumed to be 100% for calculation purposes).

1. **Calculate DMSO Volume**:

$$V_{DMSO} = \frac{30\% \; x \; 50 \; mL}{100\%} = 15 \; mL$$

2. **Measure and Mix**:
    - Measure 35 mL of sterile distilled water (50 mL total volume - 15 mL DMSO).
    - Place the water in the mixing container.
    - Slowly add 15 mL of DMSO to the water while stirring gently.

Consultation with Professionals

- **Medical Supervision**: Always consult a healthcare professional before preparing or using DMSO solutions for therapeutic purposes.
- **Pharmacist Assistance**: Pharmacists can provide guidance on dilution techniques and ensure accurate preparation.

Summary of Best Practices

- **Accuracy**: Use precise measuring tools to ensure correct concentrations.
- **Safety**: Employ appropriate PPE and handle all chemicals with care.

- **Cleanliness**: Maintain a clean working environment to prevent contamination.

- **Documentation**: Keep records of all preparations for reference and safety compliance.

Creating Different Concentrations (99%, 90%, 80%, etc.)

Understanding Stock Solutions and Target Concentrations

When working with dimethyl sulfoxide (DMSO), it's common to begin with a high-purity stock solution, typically at 99.9% concentration. Creating solutions of lower concentrations involves accurately diluting the stock solution with an appropriate solvent to achieve the desired percentage. Precise dilution is essential for ensuring both the safety and effectiveness of the resulting solution.

Fundamental Dilution Equation

The key equation used for calculating dilutions is:

$$C1 \; x \; V1 = C2 \; x \; V2$$

Where:

- C1 = Concentration of the stock solution (%)

- V1 = Volume of the stock solution required (mL)

- C2 = Desired concentration of the diluted solution (%)

- V2 = Final total volume of the diluted solution (mL)

This equation ensures that the amount of DMSO remains constant before and after dilution.

Step-by-Step Procedures for Preparing Specific Concentrations

Example 1: Preparing a 90% DMSO Solution

Objective: Prepare 100 mL of a 90% DMSO solution from a 99.9% stock solution.

Calculations:

1. **Determine Known Values:**

    o   C1 = 99.9%

    o   C2 = 90%

    o   V2 = 100 mL

2. **Calculate V1V_1V1:**

$$V_1 = \frac{C_2 \; x \; V_2}{C_1} = \frac{90\% \; x \; 100 \; mL}{99\%} \approx 90 \; mL$$

3. **Calculate Volume of Diluent (VdiluentV_{\text{diluent}}Vdiluent):**

$$V_{DILUENT} = V_2 - V_1 = 100 \; mL - 90.09 \; mL = 9.91 \; mL$$

Procedure:

- Measure **90.09 mL** of 99.9% DMSO using a graduated cylinder.

- Measure **9.91 mL** of sterile distilled water or appropriate diluent.

- Slowly add the DMSO to the diluent while stirring gently.

- Mix thoroughly until a homogeneous solution is achieved.

Example 2: Preparing an 80% DMSO Solution

Objective: Prepare 50 mL of an 80% DMSO solution from a 99.9% stock solution.

Calculations:

1. **Determine Known Values:**

   o   C1 = 99.9%

   o   C2 = 80%

   o   V2 = 50 mL

2. **Calculate V1V_1V1:**

$$V_1 = \frac{80\% \; x \; 50 \; mL}{99,9\%} \approx 40.04 \; mL$$

3. **Calculate VdiluentV_{\text{diluent}}Vdiluent:**

$$V_{DILUENT} = 50 \; mL - 40.04 \; mL = 9.96 \; mL$$

Procedure:

- Measure **40.04 mL** of 99.9% DMSO.

- Measure **9.96 mL** of sterile distilled water.

- Add DMSO to the diluent slowly, stirring continuously.

- Mix until the solution is uniform.

Example 3: Preparing a 60% DMSO Solution

Objective: Prepare 200 mL of a 60% DMSO solution from a 99.9% stock solution.

Calculations:

1. **Determine Known Values:**

   o   C1 = 99.9%

   o   C2 = 60%

   o   V2 = 200 m

2. **Calculate V1V_1V1:**

$$V_1 = \frac{60\% \; x \; 200 \; mL}{99,9\%} \approx 120.12 \; mL$$

3. **Calculate VdiluentV_{\text{diluent}}Vdiluent:**

$$V_{DILUENT} = 200 \; mL - 120.12 \; mL = 79.88 \; mL$$

Procedure:

- Measure **120.12 mL** of 99.9% DMSO.

- Measure **79.88 mL** of sterile distilled water.

- Gradually add the DMSO to the diluent with gentle stirring.

- Ensure complete mixing for a consistent solution.

Creating a Dilution Chart for Quick Reference

For ease of preparation, the following chart summarizes the volumes needed to prepare 100 mL of various DMSO concentrations from a 99.9% stock solution:

Desired Concentration (% DMSO)	Volume of Stock DMSO (mL)	Volume of Diluent (mL)
90	90.09	9.91
80	80.08	19.92
70	70.07	29.93
60	60.06	39.94
50	50.05	49.95
40	40.04	59.96
30	30.03	69.97
20	20.02	79.98
10	10.01	89.99

Note: Adjust volumes proportionally for different total volumes.

Best Practices for Accurate Dilution

- **Precision in Measurement:** Use calibrated measuring devices such as volumetric flasks, pipettes, or syringes for accurate volume determination.

- **Mixing Order:** Always add DMSO to the diluent to better control the exothermic reaction and ensure safety.

- **Temperature Control:** Perform dilutions at room temperature and allow the solution to cool if any heat is generated during mixing.

- **Avoiding Contamination:** Ensure all equipment is clean and free from contaminants. Use sterile diluents when necessary.

- **Labeling:** Clearly label all prepared solutions with the concentration, date of preparation, and expiration date.

Handling Exothermic Reactions

The mixing of DMSO with water is exothermic and can release heat:

- **Mitigation Techniques:**
  - Add DMSO slowly to the diluent with continuous stirring.
  - For larger volumes or higher concentrations, consider using an ice bath to dissipate heat.
  - Allow the solution to reach ambient temperature before use.

Safety Considerations

- **Personal Protective Equipment (PPE):**
  - Wear nitrile or latex gloves to prevent skin absorption.
  - Use safety goggles to protect eyes from splashes.
  - Wear a lab coat or apron.

- **Ventilation:** Conduct dilutions in a well-ventilated area to avoid inhalation of vapors.

- **Material Compatibility:** Use glass or compatible plastics like polypropylene; avoid materials that may react with DMSO.

Storage of Prepared Solutions

- **Container Selection:** Store diluted solutions in airtight, amber glass bottles to protect from light and moisture.

- **Storage Conditions:** Keep in a cool, dry place away from direct sunlight.

- **Shelf Life:** Follow guidelines on the stability of diluted solutions; some may require refrigeration or have limited shelf lives.

Documentation and Quality Assurance

- **Record-Keeping:** Maintain detailed records of all dilutions, including calculations, batch numbers, and any observations during preparation.

- **Quality Checks:** Periodically verify the concentration of stored solutions, especially if they are to be used over extended periods.

Practical Applications of Various Concentrations

- **99% DMSO:** Generally used as a stock solution; not recommended for direct application due to potential for irritation.

- **90% DMSO:** Used in specialized medical settings under professional supervision.

- **80% DMSO:** Employed for conditions requiring deep penetration, such as severe musculoskeletal issues.

- **70% DMSO and Below:** Commonly used for topical applications, balancing efficacy with reduced risk of irritation.

3.3.2 Dilution Charts and Calculations

Accurate preparation of dimethyl sulfoxide (DMSO) solutions at specific concentrations is essential for ensuring both the safety and efficacy of therapeutic applications. Dilution charts and systematic calculations provide a practical framework for quickly determining the volumes required to achieve desired concentrations from a stock solution. This section presents comprehensive dilution charts and elaborates on the mathematical principles underlying dilution calculations, facilitating precise and reliable preparation of DMSO solutions.

Importance of Dilution Charts

- **Efficiency**: Dilution charts offer a quick reference, reducing the time needed for calculations.

- **Accuracy**: Standardized charts minimize errors that can occur with manual calculations.

- **Safety**: Ensuring correct concentrations helps prevent adverse effects associated with improper dosing.

Understanding Dilution Principles

The process of diluting a concentrated solution involves adding a solvent to decrease the concentration of the solute. The fundamental principle is that the amount of solute remains constant before and after dilution. The key variables involved are:

- C_{STOCK}: Concentration of the stock (initial) solution.

- V_{STOCK}: Volume of the stock solution used.

- C_{FINAL}: Desired concentration of the final diluted solution.

- V_{FINAL}: Total volume of the final solution after dilution.

The relationship among these variables is expressed by the dilution equation:

$$C_{STOCK} \times V_{STOCK} = C_{FINAL} \times V_{FINAL}$$

This equation ensures the conservation of mass of the solute (DMSO in this case) during the dilution process.

Creating a Comprehensive Dilution Chart

A dilution chart serves as a practical tool for determining the volumes of stock solution and diluent required to prepare various concentrations. Below is an example of a dilution chart for preparing DMSO solutions from a 99.9% stock solution.

Table 3.1: Volumes Required to Prepare 100 mL of DMSO Solutions from a 99.9% Stock Solution

Desired Final Concentration (% DMSO)	Volume of 99.9% DMSO (mL)	Volume of Diluent (mL)
90	90.09	9.91
80	80.08	19.92
70	70.07	29.93
60	60.06	39.94
50	50.05	49.95
40	40.04	59.96
30	30.03	69.97
20	20.02	79.98
10	10.01	89.99
5	5.00	95.00
1	1.00	99.00

Note: Volumes are rounded to two decimal places for practicality.

Utilizing the Dilution Chart

To prepare a specific concentration:

1. **Identify the Desired Concentration**: Locate the target concentration in the first column.

2. **Determine Volumes**:

   o **Volume of Stock DMSO**: Use the corresponding value in the second column.

   o **Volume of Diluent**: Use the corresponding value in the third column.

3. **Measure and Mix**:

   o Accurately measure the specified volumes using appropriate equipment.

   o Add the DMSO to the diluent slowly while stirring to ensure thorough mixing.

Customizing Dilution Charts for Different Volumes

The provided dilution chart is based on preparing 100 mL of the final solution. To adjust for different total volumes, the volumes of stock solution and diluent can be scaled proportionally. The following formula facilitates this adjustment:

$$Adjusted\ Volume\ (\frac{Desired\ Total\ Volume}{100\ mL})\ x\ Volume\ from\ Chart$$

Example:

To prepare 250 mL of a 70% DMSO solution:

1. **Find the Volumes for 100 mL:**

   o Volume of DMSO: 70.07 mL

   o Volume of Diluent: 29.93 mL

2. **Calculate Adjusted Volumes:**

   o Volume of DMSO:

$$\left(\frac{250 \ mL}{100 \ mL} \right) x \ 70.07mL = 175.18 \ mL$$

   o Volume of Diluent: (250 mL100 mL)×29.93 mL=74.83 mL\left(\frac{250 \text{ mL}}{100 \text{ mL}} \right) \times 29.93 \text{ mL} = 74.83 \text{ mL}(100 mL250 mL)×29.93 mL=74.83 mL

3. **Procedure:**

   o Measure **175.18 mL** of 99.9% DMSO.

   o Measure **74.83 mL** of diluent.

   o Combine as per standard mixing protocols.

Calculating Dilutions Without a Chart

In situations where a dilution chart is unavailable, calculations can be performed manually using the dilution equation.

General Steps:

1. **Identify Known Variables:**

   o C_{STOCK}Cstock : Concentration of the stock solution.

   o C_{FINAL}Cfinal: Desired final concentration.

   o V_{FINAL}: Desired final total volume.

2. **Rearrange the Dilution Equation:**

$$V_{STOCK} = \frac{C_{FINAL} \ x \ V_{FINAL}}{C_{STOCK}}$$

3. **Calculate Vstock:**

4. **Determine Vdiluent:**

$$V_{DILUENT} = V_{FINAL} - V_{STOCK}$$

5. **Measure and Mix:**

   o Measure the calculated volumes accurately.

   o Follow safe mixing procedures.

Example:

Prepare 150 mL of a 25% DMSO solution from a 99.9% stock solution.

1. **Known Variables:**

   o Cstock = 99.9%

   o Cfinal = 25%

   o Vfinal = 150 mL

2. **Calculate Vstock:**

$$V_{STOCK} = \frac{25\% \times 150 \, mL}{99,9\%} \approx 37.54 \, mL$$

3. **Calculate Vdiluent:**

$$V_{DILUENT} = 150 \, mL - 37.54 = 112.46 \, mL$$

4. **Procedure:**

   o   Measure **37.54 mL** of 99.9% DMSO.

   o   Measure **112.46 mL** of diluent.

   o   Combine and mix thoroughly.

Preparing Serial Dilutions

For applications requiring very low concentrations, serial dilutions may be employed. This method involves successive dilutions to achieve the desired concentration.

Steps:

1. **Prepare an Intermediate Dilution:**

   o   Dilute the stock solution to an intermediate concentration.

2. **Perform Subsequent Dilutions:**

   o   Use the intermediate solution to prepare a further diluted solution.

3. **Repeat as Necessary:**

   o   Continue the process until the target concentration is achieved.

Example:

To prepare 100 mL of a 1% DMSO solution:

1. **First Dilution:**

   o   Prepare 10 mL of a 10% solution from 99.9% stock.

$$V_{STOCK} = \frac{10\% \times 10 \, mL}{99,9\%} \approx 1.00 \, mL$$

   o   Mix 1.00 mL of stock DMSO with 9.00 mL of diluent.

2. **Second Dilution:**

   o   Dilute the 10% solution to 1%:

$$V_{10\% \, SOLUTION} = \frac{1\% \times 100 \, mL}{99,9\%} \approx 10 \, mL$$

   o   Add 10 mL of the 10% solution to 90 mL of diluent.

Storage and Handling

Proper storage and handling of dimethyl sulfoxide (DMSO) are crucial to maintain its stability, efficacy, and safety for therapeutic applications. This section outlines the guidelines and best practices for storing and handling DMSO, emphasizing the importance of adhering to safety protocols to prevent degradation and minimize risks associated with its use.

Physical and Chemical Properties Relevant to Storage

Understanding the physical and chemical properties of DMSO informs appropriate storage conditions:

- **Hygroscopic Nature**: DMSO readily absorbs moisture from the atmosphere, which can alter its concentration and introduce impurities.

- **Freezing Point**: Pure DMSO solidifies at approximately 18.5°C (65.3°F), which is slightly below room temperature.

- **Chemical Stability**: DMSO is chemically stable under normal conditions but can decompose when exposed to strong oxidizing agents or extreme temperatures.

- **Compatibility**: It can react with certain materials, necessitating careful selection of storage containers.

Storage Conditions

Temperature Control

- **Optimal Temperature Range**: Store DMSO at controlled room temperature, ideally between 20°C and 25°C (68°F to 77°F).

- **Avoid Freezing**: Prevent temperatures from dropping below 18.5°C to avoid solidification, which can complicate handling.

- **Protection from Heat**: Do not expose DMSO to high temperatures, as excessive heat may accelerate degradation or increase pressure in sealed containers.

Protection from Light and Air

- **Light Sensitivity**: While DMSO is relatively stable to light, prolonged exposure to ultraviolet (UV) light may cause degradation; therefore, storing in amber-colored containers is recommended.

- **Air Exposure**: Minimize exposure to air to prevent absorption of atmospheric moisture and contaminants.

Humidity Control

- **Moisture Absorption**: Due to its hygroscopic nature, DMSO should be stored in airtight containers to prevent moisture uptake.

- **Desiccants**: Including desiccant packets in storage areas can help maintain low humidity levels.

Chapter 3: Methods of Application

Topical Use

Topical application of dimethyl sulfoxide (DMSO) involves applying the compound directly to the skin, where it can exert local or systemic effects. Due to its unique ability to penetrate biological membranes, DMSO serves as both a therapeutic agent and a vehicle for transdermal delivery of other substances. This section explores the scientific principles underlying the topical use of DMSO, its therapeutic applications, application techniques, and safety considerations.

Skin Preparation and Cleanliness

Proper skin preparation and cleanliness are paramount when applying dimethyl sulfoxide (DMSO) topically. Due to DMSO's unique ability to enhance the transdermal absorption of substances, meticulous attention to skin hygiene minimizes the risk of unintended systemic exposure to contaminants or pathogens. This section outlines the scientifically grounded procedures for preparing the skin prior to DMSO application to ensure both safety and therapeutic efficacy.

Importance of Skin Cleanliness in DMSO Application

DMSO's highly permeable nature allows it to act as a carrier molecule, facilitating the passage of not only therapeutic agents but also unintended substances through the stratum corneum into systemic circulation. Contaminants such as dirt, oils, residual cosmetics, microorganisms, and environmental toxins present on the skin surface can be inadvertently transported into the bloodstream when DMSO is applied. This underscores the necessity of thorough skin cleansing to prevent potential adverse effects stemming from the absorption of these substances.

Recommended Skin Cleansing Protocol

1. **Hand Hygiene**

   o **Washing Hands**: Before commencing skin preparation, the individual applying DMSO should wash their hands thoroughly with soap and warm water for at least 20 seconds to remove microorganisms and residues.

   o **Use of Gloves**: Donning disposable nitrile gloves after handwashing provides an additional barrier, preventing personal skin oils and contaminants from contacting the application site.

2. **Removal of Topical Agents and Debris**

   o **Cleansing Agents**: Use a mild, non-fragrant, and non-oily soap or cleanser to wash the application area. Harsh soaps or those containing oils, perfumes, or dyes should be avoided, as these substances can leave residues that may be absorbed.

   o **Technique**: Gently lather the cleanser over the skin using circular motions to ensure the removal of surface contaminants and sebum without causing abrasion or irritation.

3. **Rinsing**

   o **Water Temperature**: Rinse the area with lukewarm water. Extreme temperatures may alter skin permeability or cause vasodilation, affecting DMSO absorption rates.

   o **Thorough Removal**: Ensure all soap residues are completely rinsed off, as residual surfactants may interact with DMSO or facilitate unintended absorption.

4. **Drying**

   o **Method**: Pat the skin dry with a clean, lint-free towel or disposable paper towel. Avoid rubbing, which can cause micro-abrasions and increase skin permeability in an uncontrolled manner.

   o **Complete Dryness**: Ensure the skin is completely dry before applying DMSO, as residual moisture can dilute the DMSO concentration and potentially affect its efficacy and absorption profile.

5. **Avoidance of Contaminants Post-Cleansing**

o **No Topical Products**: Do not apply lotions, creams, perfumes, or other topical agents to the area after cleansing and before DMSO application.

o **Environmental Exposure**: Minimize exposure of the cleansed area to environmental contaminants by proceeding promptly with DMSO application in a clean environment.

Application Techniques

Effective application of dimethyl sulfoxide (DMSO) is essential to maximize its therapeutic benefits while minimizing potential adverse effects. This section provides a detailed overview of the recommended techniques for topical application of DMSO, emphasizing scientific principles and best practices.

Selection of Appropriate DMSO Concentration

- **Therapeutic Concentrations**: Commonly used concentrations for topical DMSO range from 25% to 70%, depending on the condition being treated and individual patient tolerance.

  o **Lower Concentrations (25–50%)**: Suitable for sensitive skin areas, initial treatments, or individuals prone to irritation.

  o **Higher Concentrations (50–70%)**: Employed for more severe conditions requiring deeper penetration, provided the patient tolerates higher concentrations without significant adverse effects.

- **Customization**: Concentration should be tailored based on medical advice, considering factors such as skin sensitivity, treatment area, and specific therapeutic goals.

Preparation of the DMSO Solution

- **Dilution**: If dilution is necessary, use sterile, distilled water or a compatible solvent to achieve the desired concentration.

- **Mixing**: Combine DMSO and diluent in a clean, non-reactive container (e.g., glass or compatible plastic) using aseptic techniques.

- **Stability**: Prepare fresh solutions as needed or store diluted solutions in airtight, amber-colored containers to protect from light and contamination.

Application Materials

- **Applicators**: Use sterile, disposable materials such as cotton balls, gauze pads, or applicator brushes to apply DMSO.

- **Avoid Reusable Items**: Do not use reusable sponges or cloths, as they may harbor contaminants or retain residues from previous applications.

- **Glove Use**: Wear disposable nitrile gloves to prevent personal exposure and to avoid transferring skin oils or contaminants to the application site.

Application Procedure

1. **Positioning**: Ensure the patient is comfortably positioned to allow easy access to the treatment area without stretching or compressing the skin.

2. **Dosing**:

   o **Measured Quantity**: Use a calibrated dropper or syringe without a needle to measure the exact volume of DMSO required.

   o **Layer Thickness**: Apply a thin, even layer to the skin; excessive amounts are unnecessary and may increase the risk of irritation.

3. **Application Technique**:

   o **Gentle Application**: Apply DMSO gently to the skin using smooth strokes, avoiding vigorous rubbing that could irritate the skin.

   o **Direction**: There is no specific directional requirement; focus on even coverage.

4. **Drying Time**:

   o **Absorption Period**: Allow the DMSO to air dry completely, which typically takes 10–15 minutes, depending on the concentration and environmental conditions.

   o **Avoid Blowing or Fanning**: Do not use external means to accelerate drying, as this may introduce contaminants.

5. **Post-Application Care**:

   o **Clothing**: Once dry, the area can be covered with clean, loose-fitting clothing made of natural fibers to minimize skin irritation.

   o **Avoid Occlusive Dressings**: Do not apply airtight dressings unless specifically directed by a healthcare professional.

Frequency and Duration of Application

- **Frequency**: Application frequency varies based on the therapeutic regimen but commonly ranges from one to three times daily.

- **Duration**: Treatment duration should be determined by a healthcare provider, considering the condition's response and any side effects.

- **Monitoring**: Regularly assess the treatment area for signs of improvement or adverse reactions.

Special Considerations for Sensitive Areas

- **Facial Application**:

  o **Lower Concentrations**: Use diluted DMSO (e.g., 10–25%) to minimize the risk of irritation.

  o **Avoid Contact with Eyes**: Exercise extreme caution to prevent DMSO from entering the eyes, which could cause irritation or injury.

- **Mucous Membranes**:

  o **Medical Supervision Required**: Application to mucous membranes should only be performed under professional guidance due to increased absorption and sensitivity.

Managing Adverse Reactions

- **Skin Irritation**:

  o **Signs**: Redness, itching, burning, or rash may indicate irritation.

  o **Actions**: Reduce concentration, decrease application frequency, or discontinue use as appropriate.

- **Allergic Reactions**:

  o **Symptoms**: Hives, swelling, or severe itching may suggest an allergic response.

  o **Immediate Care**: Discontinue use and seek medical attention if severe reactions occur.

Hygiene and Safety Practices

- **Handwashing**:

  o **Before and After**: Wash hands thoroughly before donning gloves and after removing them post-application.

- **Avoiding Cross-Contamination**:

  o **Single-Use Applicators**: Discard applicators after each use to prevent contamination.

  o **Separate Containers**: Do not dip used applicators back into the DMSO container.

- **Environmental Cleanliness**:

- o **Clean Workspace**: Perform applications in a clean area to minimize environmental contaminants.

- o **Surface Protection**: Use disposable pads or barriers to protect surfaces from spills or drips.

Disposal of Materials

- **Applicators and Gloves**:

  - o **Proper Disposal**: Discard used materials in accordance with local regulations for medical waste.

- **Spill Management**:

  - o **Immediate Clean-Up**: Wipe up any spills promptly using disposable absorbent materials.

  - o **Waste Disposal**: Dispose of cleaning materials appropriately to prevent environmental contamination.

Record-Keeping and Monitoring

- **Treatment Logs**:

  - o **Documentation**: Keep a detailed record of application dates, times, concentrations used, and any observed effects.

- **Progress Assessment**:

  - o **Regular Evaluation**: Assess the efficacy of treatment and adjust the regimen as necessary in consultation with a healthcare provider.

Patient Education

- **Instructions**:

  - o **Clear Guidance**: Provide written and verbal instructions on application techniques, safety precautions, and what to expect during treatment.

- **Signs of Complications**:

  - o **Awareness**: Educate patients on recognizing adverse reactions and the importance of reporting them promptly.

Legal and Ethical Considerations

- **Scope of Practice**:

  - o **Professional Standards**: Ensure that application techniques align with medical guidelines and regulatory requirements.

- **Informed Consent**:

  - o **Patient Agreement**: Obtain informed consent after discussing potential risks and benefits of topical DMSO therapy.

Oral Ingestion

Oral ingestion of dimethyl sulfoxide (DMSO) involves consuming the compound by mouth with the intention of achieving systemic therapeutic effects. While DMSO is primarily recognized for its topical applications and as a pharmaceutical solvent, its oral use has been explored in both experimental settings and alternative medicine practices. This section examines the scientific evidence surrounding oral ingestion of DMSO, including its pharmacokinetics, potential therapeutic applications, safety concerns, and regulatory status.

4.2.1 Pharmacokinetics of Oral DMSO

Absorption

When DMSO is administered orally, it is rapidly absorbed through the gastrointestinal (GI) tract. The compound's small molecular size and high polarity facilitate its passage across the mucosal membranes of the stomach and intestines.

- **Bioavailability**: Oral bioavailability of DMSO approaches 100%, indicating that nearly the entire administered dose enters systemic circulation.

- **Peak Plasma Concentrations**: Maximum plasma concentrations are typically reached within 2 to 4 hours post-ingestion.

Distribution

After absorption, DMSO is distributed widely throughout the body:

- **Tissue Penetration**: It crosses biological membranes, including the blood-brain barrier, leading to distribution in various tissues such as the liver, kidneys, lungs, and central nervous system.

- **Volume of Distribution**: DMSO exhibits a large volume of distribution, reflecting its extensive penetration into body compartments.

Metabolism

DMSO undergoes metabolism primarily in the liver:

- **Oxidation**: The major metabolic pathway involves oxidation to dimethyl sulfone ($DMSO_2$), a process mediated by hepatic enzymes.

- **Reduction**: A minor pathway reduces DMSO to dimethyl sulfide (DMS), which is responsible for the characteristic garlic-like odor on the breath and skin.

Excretion

Elimination of DMSO and its metabolites occurs via multiple routes:

- **Renal Excretion**: The majority of DMSO and $DMSO_2$ is excreted unchanged in the urine.

- **Pulmonary Excretion**: Dimethyl sulfide is exhaled through the lungs, contributing to the aforementioned odor.

- **Half-Life**: The elimination half-life of DMSO ranges from 8 to 20 hours, depending on factors such as dose and individual metabolic rates.

Potential Therapeutic Applications

Research into the oral use of DMSO has explored various potential therapeutic effects. It is important to note that much of this research is preliminary, and robust clinical evidence supporting these applications is limited.

Anti-Inflammatory and Analgesic Effects

- **Mechanism**: DMSO may exert systemic anti-inflammatory effects by inhibiting the production of pro-inflammatory cytokines and modulating immune cell function.

- **Applications**: Some studies have investigated its use in conditions such as rheumatoid arthritis and musculoskeletal pain.

Antioxidant Properties

- **Free Radical Scavenging**: DMSO's ability to neutralize reactive oxygen species suggests potential benefits in diseases associated with oxidative stress.

- **Neuroprotection**: Experimental models have examined DMSO's role in mitigating neuronal damage following ischemic events or traumatic injuries.

Cardiovascular Effects

- **Vasodilation**: DMSO may promote vasodilation, potentially improving blood flow and reducing blood pressure.

- **Cholesterol Reduction**: Limited studies have suggested possible effects on lipid profiles.

Immunomodulation

- **Autoimmune Conditions**: By modulating immune responses, DMSO has been hypothesized to have therapeutic potential in autoimmune diseases.

Safety and Toxicity Considerations

The oral ingestion of DMSO raises significant safety concerns that necessitate careful evaluation.

Gastrointestinal Irritation

- **Symptoms**: Oral DMSO may cause nausea, vomiting, diarrhea, and abdominal cramps.
- **Mucosal Irritation**: High concentrations can irritate the GI mucosa, leading to discomfort or ulceration.

Central Nervous System Effects

- **Neurotoxicity**: At high doses, DMSO has been associated with headaches, dizziness, sedation, and, in severe cases, seizures.
- **Cognitive Impairment**: Some users report difficulty concentrating or memory disturbances.

Renal and Hepatic Effects

- **Nephrotoxicity**: Animal studies have indicated potential renal damage with high-dose DMSO ingestion.
- **Hepatotoxicity**: Liver enzyme elevations have been observed, suggesting possible hepatic stress or injury.

Hematological Effects

- **Blood Disorders**: Rare cases of hemolysis and alterations in blood cell counts have been reported.

Allergic Reactions

- **Hypersensitivity**: Allergic responses, including anaphylactoid reactions, may occur in susceptible individuals.

Odor and Taste Disturbances

- **Garlic-like Odor**: Metabolism to dimethyl sulfide leads to a persistent odor on the breath and skin, which can be socially problematic.
- **Taste Alterations**: Users may experience a lingering taste disturbance.

Regulatory Status and Professional Guidelines

Lack of FDA Approval

- **United States**: The Food and Drug Administration (FDA) has not approved DMSO for oral ingestion in humans. Its approved medical use is limited to intravesical administration for interstitial cystitis.
- **Implications**: The absence of regulatory approval reflects insufficient evidence of safety and efficacy for oral use.

International Perspectives

- **Other Countries**: Regulatory agencies in most countries mirror the FDA's position, not endorsing oral DMSO for therapeutic purposes.
- **Exceptions**: Some regions may have less stringent regulations, but professional medical bodies generally advise caution.

Professional Guidelines

- **Medical Consensus**: Health professionals typically discourage oral DMSO use due to potential risks and the lack of validated clinical benefits.
- **Research Recommendations**: Further studies, including randomized controlled trials, are necessary to establish safety profiles and therapeutic efficacy.

Mixing with Juices and Other Liquids

Overview

The practice of mixing dimethyl sulfoxide (DMSO) with juices or other beverages for oral ingestion has emerged among some individuals aiming to mask its strong taste and odor or to facilitate consumption. This section examines the scientific implications of combining DMSO with various liquids, highlighting potential chemical interactions, effects on absorption, and safety concerns. It is important to note that the oral administration of DMSO is not approved by regulatory agencies due to insufficient evidence regarding its safety and efficacy.

Solubility and Chemical Compatibility

Miscibility with Aqueous Solutions

- **High Solubility in Water**: DMSO is highly miscible with water and can readily dissolve in aqueous solutions, including juices and other beverages.

- **Solvent Properties**: As a polar aprotic solvent, DMSO can dissolve both polar and nonpolar substances, potentially affecting the composition of the beverage it is mixed with.

Potential Chemical Interactions

- **Reactivity with Beverage Components**: DMSO may interact with certain compounds present in juices, such as acids, sugars, and phytochemicals. These interactions could alter the chemical structure of DMSO or the beverage components.

- **Formation of Byproducts**: Chemical reactions between DMSO and constituents of the liquid might lead to the formation of new compounds, the effects of which are not well understood.

Impact on Absorption and Pharmacokinetics

Enhanced Absorption of Beverage Constituents

- **Carrier Properties**: DMSO's ability to facilitate the transmembrane transport of molecules raises concerns that it may enhance the systemic absorption of substances present in the beverage, including additives, preservatives, or contaminants.

- **Unintended Bioavailability**: Increased absorption of certain compounds could lead to unanticipated pharmacological effects or toxicity.

Alteration of DMSO Absorption

- **Dilution Effect**: Mixing DMSO with large volumes of liquid may dilute its concentration, potentially affecting its absorption rate and peak plasma concentrations.

- **Gastrointestinal Transit Time**: The presence of food or beverages in the stomach can influence gastric emptying and intestinal transit times, thereby modifying the pharmacokinetics of DMSO.

Sensory Considerations

Taste and Odor Challenges

- **Strong Odor**: DMSO has a characteristic garlic-like odor resulting from its metabolism to dimethyl sulfide (DMS). Mixing it with juices may not effectively mask this odor.

- **Taste Masking**: While combining DMSO with flavored beverages might partially obscure its taste, the solvent properties of DMSO can alter the flavor profile of the drink, potentially leading to an unpleasant taste experience.

Patient Compliance

- **Palatability Issues**: Unpleasant taste and odor may affect adherence to any regimen involving oral DMSO, although this is secondary given the lack of approval for oral use.

Safety Concerns

Gastrointestinal Irritation

- **Irritative Potential**: The combination of DMSO with acidic juices (e.g., citrus juices) might exacerbate gastrointestinal irritation, potentially leading to discomfort or mucosal damage.

- **Concentration Variability**: Mixing DMSO with liquids without precise measurement can result in inconsistent dosing, increasing the risk of adverse effects.

Contaminant Introduction

- **Purity of Liquids**: Beverages may contain substances that, while safe under normal consumption, could pose risks when their absorption is enhanced by DMSO.

- **Alcohol Content**: Mixing DMSO with alcoholic beverages may potentiate the effects of alcohol and increase central nervous system depression.

Allergic and Hypersensitivity Reactions

- **Additives and Preservatives**: Enhanced absorption of allergens or sensitizing agents present in beverages could trigger allergic reactions.

Potential Side Effects

Overview

Oral ingestion of dimethyl sulfoxide (DMSO) can lead to a range of potential side effects due to its pharmacological actions and interactions within the body. While DMSO is primarily approved for specific medical applications such as intravesical therapy for interstitial cystitis, its oral use is not widely endorsed or thoroughly studied. This section examines the potential adverse effects associated with the oral consumption of DMSO, highlighting the importance of caution and medical supervision.

Gastrointestinal Effects

- **Mucosal Irritation**: DMSO can irritate the lining of the gastrointestinal (GI) tract, leading to symptoms such as nausea, vomiting, abdominal pain, and diarrhea. The solvent properties of DMSO may disrupt the protective mucous layer, increasing the risk of erosion or ulceration.

- **Altered GI Motility**: Some individuals may experience changes in bowel habits, including constipation or increased frequency of defecation, due to DMSO's effect on smooth muscle activity.

Neurological Effects

- **Headaches and Dizziness**: Oral DMSO ingestion has been associated with central nervous system side effects like headaches, dizziness, and lightheadedness. These symptoms may result from DMSO's vasodilatory effects or direct neural interactions.

- **Sedation and Fatigue**: Some users report feelings of sedation, lethargy, or general fatigue, potentially impacting daily activities and alertness.

- **Peripheral Neuropathy**: Although rare, there have been reports of tingling sensations or numbness in the extremities, suggesting potential effects on peripheral nerves.

Hepatic and Renal Effects

- **Liver Enzyme Elevations**: DMSO metabolism occurs predominantly in the liver. Oral ingestion may lead to transient increases in liver enzymes (e.g., AST, ALT), indicating hepatic stress or mild hepatocellular injury.

- **Renal Impairment**: The kidneys are involved in excreting DMSO and its metabolites. High doses or prolonged use may place additional strain on renal function, particularly in individuals with pre-existing kidney conditions.

Cardiovascular Effects

- **Hypotension**: DMSO's vasodilatory properties can cause a decrease in blood pressure, leading to hypotension. Symptoms may include dizziness upon standing (orthostatic hypotension), faintness, or even syncope (loss of consciousness).

- **Flushing**: Users may experience warmth or redness in the face and neck due to vasodilation of superficial blood vessels.

Dermatological Effects

- **Garlic-like Odor**: A common side effect is a strong garlic-like smell on the breath and skin. This odor results from the metabolic conversion of DMSO to dimethyl sulfide (DMS) and can persist for up to 72 hours after ingestion.

- **Skin Reactions**: Some individuals may develop rashes, itching, or other allergic skin reactions, possibly due to hypersensitivity to DMSO or its metabolites.

Respiratory Effects

- **Bronchospasm**: In susceptible individuals, particularly those with asthma or other respiratory conditions, DMSO may induce bronchospasm, leading to coughing, wheezing, or shortness of breath.

- **Respiratory Irritation**: Inhalation of DMSO vapors (from exhaled air after ingestion) can irritate the respiratory tract.

Hematological Effects

- **Coagulopathy**: DMSO may affect platelet function and coagulation pathways, potentially increasing the risk of bleeding or bruising.

- **Anemia**: There are isolated reports of anemia following oral DMSO use, possibly due to hemolysis or bone marrow suppression, although this is not well-documented.

Immunological Effects

- **Immunosuppression**: DMSO may modulate immune function, potentially leading to decreased resistance to infections.

- **Allergic Reactions**: Hypersensitivity reactions, including urticaria (hives), angioedema (swelling of deeper skin layers), and, in severe cases, anaphylaxis, have been reported.

Endocrine and Metabolic Effects

- **Hyperglycemia**: Some evidence suggests that DMSO may interfere with glucose metabolism, potentially causing elevated blood sugar levels.

- **Electrolyte Imbalances**: Gastrointestinal side effects like vomiting and diarrhea can lead to dehydration and disturbances in electrolyte balance (e.g., low potassium or sodium levels).

Reproductive Effects

- **Teratogenicity**: Animal studies have indicated potential teratogenic effects (birth defects) when DMSO is administered during pregnancy. The safety of DMSO in pregnant or breastfeeding women has not been established.

- **Fertility Concerns**: There is limited information on DMSO's effects on human fertility, but some animal studies suggest possible adverse impacts on reproductive organs.

Drug Interactions

- **Enhanced Absorption**: DMSO's carrier properties may increase the absorption of concomitant medications, potentially leading to higher plasma concentrations and increased risk of toxicity.

- **Altered Metabolism**: DMSO may inhibit or induce cytochrome P450 enzymes, affecting the metabolism of other drugs and leading to unexpected therapeutic outcomes.

Psychological Effects

- **Mood Changes**: Some users report mood swings, anxiety, or depressive symptoms, although these effects are not well-characterized and may be secondary to other systemic effects.

- **Sleep Disturbances**: Insomnia or altered sleep patterns have been observed in some individuals following oral ingestion.

Sensory Effects

- **Taste Alterations**: A persistent metallic or garlic-like taste may occur, affecting appetite and enjoyment of food.

- **Visual Disturbances**: Blurred vision or changes in visual acuity have been reported anecdotally, necessitating caution in activities requiring clear vision.

Musculoskeletal Effects

- **Muscle Cramps**: Electrolyte imbalances caused by gastrointestinal losses may lead to muscle cramps or weakness.

- **Joint Pain**: Paradoxically, while DMSO is used for its anti-inflammatory properties, some users may experience joint discomfort or exacerbation of existing musculoskeletal conditions.

Long-Term Risks

- **Carcinogenicity**: There is insufficient evidence regarding the carcinogenic potential of DMSO in humans. Long-term studies are lacking, and animal studies have yielded inconclusive results.

- **Organ Toxicity**: Chronic ingestion may lead to cumulative organ toxicity, particularly affecting the liver and kidneys.

Factors Influencing Side Effects

- **Dosage**: Higher doses are more likely to produce significant side effects. Without standardized dosing guidelines, the risk of overdose increases.

- **Duration of Use**: Prolonged use may exacerbate side effects and increase the likelihood of cumulative toxicity.

- **Individual Susceptibility**: Age, pre-existing medical conditions, genetic factors, and concurrent medication use can influence the severity and type of side effects experienced.

Monitoring and Management

- **Medical Supervision**: Regular monitoring of liver and kidney function tests, complete blood counts, and electrolyte levels is advisable if oral DMSO use is undertaken.

- **Symptom Management**: Supportive care for side effects may include antiemetics for nausea, antihistamines for allergic reactions, and fluids for dehydration.

- **Discontinuation**: If significant adverse effects occur, cessation of DMSO use is recommended, along with appropriate medical intervention.

Intravenous Use (Under Medical Supervision)

Overview

Intravenous administration of dimethyl sulfoxide (DMSO) involves the direct infusion of the compound into the bloodstream under strict medical supervision. While DMSO is primarily recognized for its topical applications and as a cryoprotectant in stem cell preservation, its intravenous use has been explored in specific clinical settings. This section examines the scientific evidence, potential therapeutic applications, pharmacokinetics, safety considerations, and regulatory status associated with intravenous DMSO administration.

Pharmacokinetics of Intravenous DMSO

Absorption and Distribution

- **Immediate Bioavailability**: Intravenous infusion of DMSO results in 100% bioavailability, allowing for rapid systemic distribution.

- **Tissue Penetration**: DMSO readily crosses biological membranes, including the blood-brain barrier, due to its low molecular weight and amphiphilic properties.

- **Volume of Distribution**: Exhibits a large volume of distribution, indicating extensive tissue uptake beyond the vascular compartment.

Metabolism

- **Primary Pathways**: Metabolized predominantly in the liver through oxidation to dimethyl sulfone ($DMSO_2$) and reduction to dimethyl sulfide (DMS).

- **Enzymatic Involvement**: Cytochrome P450 enzymes facilitate the metabolic processes.

- **Metabolite Activity**: $DMSO_2$ retains some biological activity, whereas DMS is responsible for the characteristic garlic-like odor.

Excretion

- **Renal Elimination**: Majority of DMSO and its metabolites are excreted via the kidneys.

- **Pulmonary Excretion**: DMS is eliminated through exhalation, contributing to breath odor.

- **Half-Life**: The elimination half-life ranges from 8 to 20 hours, varying with individual metabolic rates and renal function.

Potential Therapeutic Applications

Use in Hematopoietic Stem Cell Transplantation

- **Cryoprotectant Role**: DMSO is employed to preserve stem cells during freezing; upon thawing, the DMSO-containing cell product is infused intravenously.

- **Clinical Significance**: Essential in autologous and allogeneic stem cell transplants for hematological malignancies and disorders.

Experimental Therapies

- **Cerebral Edema Management**: Investigated for reducing intracranial pressure in traumatic brain injury and stroke due to its osmotic properties.

- **Anti-Inflammatory Effects**: Explored as a systemic anti-inflammatory agent in conditions like severe rheumatoid arthritis.

- **Antioxidant Properties**: Studied for mitigating oxidative stress in various pathologies, including ischemia-reperfusion injury.

Safety and Adverse Effects

Hemodynamic Changes

- **Hypotension**: Rapid infusion can cause vasodilation leading to decreased blood pressure; monitoring is crucial.

- **Cardiac Arrhythmias**: Potential for arrhythmias necessitates electrocardiographic monitoring during infusion.

Hypersensitivity Reactions

- **Anaphylactoid Responses**: Rare but serious reactions may include urticaria, bronchospasm, and hypotension.

- **Management**: Pre-medication with antihistamines and corticosteroids may be considered; emergency equipment should be readily available.

Neurological Effects

- **Headache and Dizziness**: Common transient side effects due to vascular changes or direct neural effects.

- **Seizure Risk**: High doses have been associated with an increased risk of seizures in susceptible individuals.

Renal and Hepatic Considerations

- **Nephrotoxicity**: DMSO can cause osmotic diuresis; caution in patients with impaired renal function.

- **Hepatotoxicity**: Liver enzyme elevations may occur; liver function tests should be monitored.

Gastrointestinal Symptoms

- **Nausea and Vomiting**: Frequent side effects that can be managed with antiemetic medications.

- **Abdominal Discomfort**: May result from vasodilatory effects on the gastrointestinal vasculature.

Odor-Related Effects

- **Breath and Body Odor**: Metabolism to DMS leads to a noticeable garlic-like smell, which may persist for several hours post-infusion.

Administration Protocols

Medical Supervision

- **Qualified Personnel**: Only trained healthcare professionals should administer intravenous DMSO.

- **Monitoring Parameters**: Continuous monitoring of vital signs, oxygen saturation, and cardiac rhythm is essential.

Dosage and Infusion Rate

- **Individualized Dosing**: Based on body weight, clinical condition, and specific therapeutic goals.

- **Controlled Infusion**: Infusion rates should be slow to minimize adverse effects; typical rates are determined by institutional protocols.

Pre-Infusion Assessment

- **Baseline Evaluation**: Assess renal and hepatic function, electrolyte levels, and cardiovascular status.

- **Allergy History**: Document any prior hypersensitivity reactions to DMSO or related compounds.

Post-Infusion Care

- **Observation Period**: Patients should be monitored for delayed reactions following infusion.

- **Symptom Management**: Address any side effects promptly with appropriate interventions.

Regulatory Status

Approved Uses

- **Stem Cell Infusions**: The only widely accepted intravenous exposure to DMSO in humans occurs during the infusion of cryopreserved stem cell products.

Investigational Applications

- **Clinical Trials**: Intravenous DMSO is used experimentally under approved research protocols; patients should be enrolled in formal studies with ethical oversight.

Regulatory Guidelines

- **FDA Position**: In the United States, the FDA has not approved intravenous DMSO for general therapeutic use beyond its role in stem cell transplantation.

- **International Perspectives**: Regulatory stances vary by country but generally align with caution due to limited clinical evidence.

DMSO in Combination with Other Substances

Introduction

Dimethyl sulfoxide (DMSO) is renowned for its ability to enhance the absorption and efficacy of various therapeutic agents. By serving as a solvent and penetration enhancer, DMSO can facilitate the delivery of drugs and other bioactive compounds across biological membranes. This section delves into the scientific principles, therapeutic applications, and safety considerations of using DMSO in combination with other substances.

Mechanisms of Enhanced Delivery

Solvent Properties

- **Broad Solubility Spectrum**: DMSO can dissolve both hydrophilic and hydrophobic substances due to its amphiphilic nature. This property enables the formulation of homogeneous mixtures with a wide range of compounds.

- **Stabilization of Molecules**: It can stabilize certain drugs in solution, preventing degradation and preserving therapeutic activity.

Membrane Interaction

- **Alteration of Membrane Fluidity**: DMSO interacts with lipid components of cell membranes, transiently increasing permeability without causing permanent damage.

- **Facilitation of Transdermal Transport**: By disrupting the stratum corneum barrier, DMSO enhances the transdermal penetration of co-administered agents.

Modulation of Pharmacokinetics

- **Increased Absorption Rate**: DMSO can accelerate the uptake of drugs by increasing their concentration gradient across membranes.

- **Enhanced Bioavailability**: Improved absorption can lead to higher systemic levels of the drug, potentially enhancing efficacy.

Therapeutic Applications

Anti-Inflammatory Agents

- **Nonsteroidal Anti-Inflammatory Drugs (NSAIDs)**: Combining DMSO with NSAIDs like diclofenac or ketoprofen can enhance their penetration to inflamed tissues, providing more effective pain relief.

- **Corticosteroids**: DMSO can facilitate the delivery of topical steroids used in dermatological conditions, potentially improving outcomes in psoriasis and eczema.

Antimicrobial Therapies

- **Antibiotics**: The addition of DMSO can improve the penetration of topical antibiotics into infected tissues, aiding in the treatment of bacterial skin infections.

- **Antifungal Agents**: DMSO enhances the absorption of antifungal medications like clotrimazole, benefiting conditions such as athlete's foot and nail fungus.

Antiviral Treatments

- **Herpes Simplex Virus (HSV)**: DMSO has been used experimentally to enhance the delivery of antiviral agents like acyclovir, aiming to reduce the duration and severity of outbreaks.

Chemotherapy

- **Anticancer Drugs**: In laboratory settings, DMSO has been employed to increase the uptake of chemotherapeutic agents by cancer cells, potentially improving their cytotoxic effects.

Natural Compounds and Nutraceuticals

- **Herbal Extracts**: DMSO can enhance the absorption of bioactive components from herbal remedies, such as curcumin from turmeric or allicin from garlic.

- **Vitamins and Minerals**: It may facilitate the transdermal delivery of certain vitamins, like vitamin C or B12, though clinical evidence is limited.

Formulation and Compatibility

Chemical Stability

- **Avoiding Degradation**: It's crucial to ensure that DMSO does not chemically react with the combined substance, which could inactivate the drug or produce harmful byproducts.

- **pH Considerations**: The pH of the DMSO mixture should be compatible with both the drug and the application site to prevent irritation or reduced efficacy.

Concentration Optimization

- **Effective Dosing**: Determining the optimal concentrations of DMSO and the co-administered substance is essential for maximizing therapeutic benefits while minimizing side effects.

- **Solubility Limits**: The solubility of the drug in DMSO must be sufficient to create a stable solution or suspension.

Safety Considerations

Potential Adverse Effects

- **Increased Toxicity Risk**: Enhanced absorption may lead to higher systemic concentrations of the drug, potentially causing toxicity.

- **Skin Reactions**: Combining DMSO with other substances can increase the likelihood of skin irritation, redness, or allergic responses.

Precautionary Measures

- **Quality of Ingredients**: Use only pharmaceutical-grade DMSO and high-purity drugs to avoid introducing contaminants.

- **Allergy Testing**: A patch test may be advisable to check for hypersensitivity reactions before widespread application.

- **Medical Oversight**: Healthcare professionals should supervise the use of DMSO combinations to monitor for adverse effects and adjust treatment as necessary.

Drug Interactions and Contraindications

Pharmacodynamic Interactions

- **Synergistic Effects**: While synergism can enhance therapeutic outcomes, it may also increase the risk of adverse reactions.

- **Antagonistic Effects**: DMSO might interfere with the action of certain drugs, reducing their effectiveness.

Contraindications

- **Pregnancy and Lactation**: The safety of DMSO combinations during pregnancy or breastfeeding is not well-established; therefore, use is generally discouraged.

- **Pre-existing Conditions**: Individuals with liver or kidney impairment should exercise caution due to altered metabolism and excretion.

Essential Oils

Introduction

The combination of dimethyl sulfoxide (DMSO) with essential oils has gained attention due to the potential synergistic effects on therapeutic outcomes. Essential oils are concentrated extracts derived from plants, containing volatile aromatic compounds with various biological activities, including anti-inflammatory, antimicrobial, and analgesic properties. This section explores the scientific basis, potential benefits, formulation considerations, and safety aspects of using DMSO in conjunction with essential oils for therapeutic applications.

Mechanisms of Enhanced Delivery

DMSO as a Penetration Enhancer

- **Stratum Corneum Modification**: DMSO disrupts the intercellular lipid structure of the stratum corneum, the outermost layer of the skin, increasing its permeability. This modification facilitates the transdermal absorption of essential oil constituents, which are typically lipophilic.

- **Solvent Properties**: DMSO's ability to dissolve both polar and non-polar compounds allows it to act as a carrier for a wide range of essential oil components, enhancing their penetration into deeper skin layers and systemic circulation.

Synergistic Therapeutic Effects

- **Potentiation of Biological Activity**: The combination may amplify the therapeutic effects of essential oils by ensuring higher local concentrations at the target site. DMSO's anti-inflammatory and antioxidant properties could complement those of certain essential oils.

Therapeutic Applications

Anti-Inflammatory and Analgesic Effects

- **Musculoskeletal Conditions**: Essential oils like peppermint (Mentha × piperita), eucalyptus (Eucalyptus globulus), and lavender (Lavandula angustifolia) possess anti-inflammatory and analgesic properties. When combined with DMSO, they may provide enhanced relief in conditions such as arthritis, muscle strains, and joint pain.

- **Neuropathic Pain**: Oils containing compounds like menthol or eugenol might benefit from DMSO-facilitated delivery, potentially improving outcomes in neuropathic pain management.

Antimicrobial and Antifungal Activity

- **Skin Infections**: Tea tree oil (Melaleuca alternifolia) and oregano oil (Origanum vulgare) exhibit antimicrobial effects against a variety of pathogens. DMSO may enhance their penetration to affected areas, improving efficacy in treating bacterial and fungal skin infections.

Dermatological Applications

- **Wound Healing**: Certain essential oils have properties that support wound healing and tissue regeneration. DMSO's ability to improve absorption could aid in delivering these benefits more effectively to damaged skin.

Formulation Considerations

Concentration and Dilution

- **Essential Oil Dilution**: Essential oils are potent and often require dilution to safe concentrations (usually 1–5%) in a carrier oil before application. Combining them with DMSO necessitates careful calculation to avoid skin irritation or systemic toxicity.

- **DMSO Concentration**: Optimal DMSO concentrations for transdermal delivery typically range from 25% to 50%. Higher concentrations may increase permeability but also raise the risk of adverse skin reactions.

Compatibility and Stability

- **Chemical Stability**: The formulation should ensure that essential oil constituents remain chemically stable in the presence of DMSO. Oxidation or degradation of active compounds could reduce efficacy or produce unwanted byproducts.

- **Physical Stability**: The mixture should remain homogeneous without phase separation. Emulsifiers or solubilizers might be required to maintain stability over time.

pH and Osmolarity

- **Skin Tolerance**: The pH of the final preparation should be compatible with skin physiology (typically pH 4.5–6.5) to minimize irritation. DMSO and essential oils should not significantly alter the pH beyond this range.

Safety Considerations

Skin Irritation and Sensitization

- **Potential for Irritation**: Both DMSO and essential oils can cause skin irritation or allergic reactions, particularly at higher concentrations. Symptoms may include redness, itching, burning sensations, or dermatitis.

- **Patch Testing**: Prior to widespread application, a patch test on a small skin area is advisable to assess individual sensitivity to the formulation.

Systemic Toxicity

- **Enhanced Absorption Risks**: DMSO may increase systemic absorption of essential oil components, potentially leading to toxicity, especially with oils containing potent compounds like thujone or phenols.

- **Dose Limitation**: Careful control of both DMSO and essential oil dosages is crucial to prevent systemic side effects.

Contraindications

- **Pregnancy and Breastfeeding**: Some essential oils are contraindicated during pregnancy or lactation due to potential teratogenic or toxic effects. Enhanced absorption via DMSO could increase these risks.

- **Pediatric Use**: Children's skin is more permeable, and they may be more susceptible to toxicity. Use in pediatric populations should be approached with caution and under professional guidance.

Application Techniques

Preparation

- **Formulation**: Combine pharmaceutical-grade DMSO with high-quality, pure essential oils. Ensure accurate measurement of each component to achieve the desired concentrations.

- **Mixing**: Use non-reactive containers (e.g., glass) and stir gently to create a uniform mixture.

Application

- **Skin Preparation**: Clean the application area thoroughly to remove contaminants that could be carried into the skin by DMSO.

- **Method**: Apply a small amount of the mixture using a sterile applicator, avoiding excessive quantities.

- **Frequency**: Follow guidelines provided by a healthcare professional, typically not exceeding two to three applications per day.

Castor Oil

Introduction

Castor oil, derived from the seeds of *Ricinus communis*, is a triglyceride rich in ricinoleic acid, a monounsaturated fatty acid with notable therapeutic properties. It has been used traditionally for its anti-inflammatory, analgesic, and laxative effects. Combining dimethyl sulfoxide (DMSO) with castor oil has gained interest due to the potential synergistic effects on enhancing therapeutic outcomes. This section explores the scientific rationale, potential benefits, formulation strategies, and safety considerations of using DMSO in conjunction with castor oil.

Mechanisms of Interaction

Enhanced Transdermal Delivery

- **Solvent and Carrier Properties of DMSO**: DMSO acts as a penetration enhancer by altering the permeability of biological membranes. It can disrupt the stratum corneum lipid structure, facilitating the transdermal transport of compounds.

- **Castor Oil's Emollient Effect**: Castor oil possesses skin-conditioning properties that can soften and hydrate the skin, potentially aiding in the absorption of co-applied substances.

- **Synergistic Penetration**: The combination of DMSO and castor oil may result in improved dermal penetration of bioactive constituents due to the solvent action of DMSO and the occlusive effect of castor oil.

Pharmacological Complementarity

- **Anti-Inflammatory Actions**: DMSO exhibits anti-inflammatory properties by scavenging free radicals and modulating prostaglandin synthesis. Castor oil's ricinoleic acid has been shown to inhibit inflammatory mediators like prostaglandin E2.

- **Analgesic Effects**: Both agents may contribute to pain relief through different mechanisms, potentially offering enhanced analgesia when used together.

Therapeutic Applications

Musculoskeletal Disorders

- **Arthritis and Joint Pain**: The combination may alleviate symptoms associated with osteoarthritis and rheumatoid arthritis by reducing inflammation and pain in affected joints.

- **Muscle Strains and Sprains**: Topical application could assist in relieving muscle soreness and promoting recovery after physical exertion.

Dermatological Conditions

- **Wound Healing**: Castor oil's moisturizing effect may support skin regeneration, while DMSO's antimicrobial properties could reduce infection risk.

- **Skin Infections**: The antimicrobial activity of ricinoleic acid, enhanced by DMSO's penetration, might be beneficial in treating minor skin infections.

Gastrointestinal Applications

- **Transdermal Laxative Effect**: While castor oil is traditionally used orally as a laxative, transdermal application with DMSO is not common and requires further research to establish efficacy and safety.

Formulation Strategies

Concentration Optimization

- **DMSO Concentration**: Typically used at concentrations ranging from 25% to 70% for topical applications, depending on tolerance and therapeutic needs.

- **Castor Oil Ratio**: The proportion of castor oil must be balanced to maintain an appropriate viscosity and ensure effective skin absorption without causing excessive greasiness.

Preparation Method

- **Homogeneous Mixing**: Due to the differing polarities, creating a stable mixture may require the use of emulsifiers or thorough mechanical mixing to achieve a uniform formulation.

- **Stability Considerations**: The formulation should remain stable over time without phase separation. Antioxidants may be added to prevent oxidation of fatty acids in castor oil.

Application Form

- **Creams and Ointments**: Incorporating both agents into a cream or ointment base can facilitate ease of application and enhance skin contact time.

- **Patches or Wraps**: Using occlusive dressings may increase absorption but should be approached cautiously due to potential irritation.

Safety and Toxicity

Skin Irritation and Sensitivity

- **DMSO-Related Effects**: Potential for skin irritation, redness, and dermatitis, especially at higher concentrations.

- **Castor Oil Allergies**: Although rare, some individuals may exhibit allergic reactions to castor oil, necessitating a patch test prior to widespread use.

- **Combined Effects**: The penetration-enhancing property of DMSO could increase the likelihood of irritation from castor oil constituents.

Systemic Absorption Risks

- **Enhanced Drug Delivery**: DMSO may facilitate systemic absorption of castor oil components and any impurities, which could lead to unintended systemic effects.

- **Contaminant Introduction**: Ensuring the use of high-quality, pure castor oil is crucial to prevent the introduction of harmful substances.

Contraindications and Precautions

- **Pregnancy and Lactation**: Due to the potential for systemic absorption and the laxative effect of ricinoleic acid, use during pregnancy and breastfeeding is not recommended without medical advice.

- **Pre-existing Skin Conditions**: Individuals with dermatological disorders should consult a healthcare professional before use.

Practical Application Guidelines

Skin Preparation

- **Clean Application Site**: Ensure the skin is free from contaminants to prevent unintended absorption of harmful substances.

- **Avoiding Broken Skin**: Do not apply to open wounds or severely damaged skin unless directed by a healthcare professional.

Application Technique

- **Dosage Control**: Apply a thin layer to the affected area, avoiding excessive amounts that could increase absorption risks.

- **Frequency**: Use as directed by a healthcare provider, typically not exceeding two to three times daily.

Monitoring and Follow-Up

- **Adverse Reaction Observation**: Monitor for signs of skin irritation or allergic responses.

- **Effectiveness Assessment**: Evaluate therapeutic outcomes to determine the necessity for continued use or adjustments.

MSM (Methylsulfonylmethane)

Introduction

Methylsulfonylmethane (MSM) is an organosulfur compound naturally found in small amounts in fruits, vegetables, grains, and animal products. It is commonly used as a dietary supplement for its potential anti-inflammatory, antioxidant, and analgesic properties. Combining dimethyl sulfoxide (DMSO) with MSM may enhance therapeutic outcomes due to their complementary mechanisms of action and structural similarities. This section explores the scientific basis, therapeutic applications, formulation strategies, and safety considerations of using DMSO in conjunction with MSM.

Chemical Relationship Between DMSO and MSM

Structural Similarities

- **Molecular Composition**: Both DMSO (C_2H_6OS) and MSM ($C_2H_6O_2S$) share similar molecular structures, differing primarily by an additional oxygen atom in MSM.

- **Metabolic Conversion**: DMSO is metabolized in the body to form MSM, suggesting that combined administration could potentially amplify the therapeutic effects attributed to sulfur-containing compounds.

Sulfur Donor Properties

- **Biological Significance of Sulfur**: Sulfur is essential for the synthesis of amino acids like methionine and cysteine, which are critical for protein synthesis, enzyme function, and antioxidant defense systems.

- **Role of MSM**: As a sulfur donor, MSM contributes to the maintenance of connective tissue integrity and antioxidant capacity.

Mechanisms of Action

Anti-Inflammatory Effects

- **Cytokine Modulation**: MSM has been shown to inhibit pro-inflammatory cytokines such as interleukin-6 (IL-6) and tumor necrosis factor-alpha (TNF-α).

- **Inhibition of NF-κB Pathway**: Both MSM and DMSO may suppress the nuclear factor kappa-light-chain-enhancer of activated B cells (NF-κB) signaling pathway, which plays a key role in regulating inflammatory responses.

Antioxidant Activity

- **Reactive Oxygen Species Scavenging**: MSM can neutralize reactive oxygen species (ROS), reducing oxidative stress and cellular damage.

- **Enhancement of Glutathione Levels**: MSM may boost the synthesis of glutathione, a vital intracellular antioxidant.

Joint and Connective Tissue Support

- **Cartilage Preservation**: MSM may inhibit cartilage-degrading enzymes like collagenase, promoting joint health.

- **Collagen Synthesis**: Sulfur from MSM is essential for collagen formation, aiding in the maintenance of connective tissues.

Therapeutic Applications

Osteoarthritis and Joint Disorders

- **Symptom Relief**: Clinical studies indicate that MSM supplementation can reduce pain, stiffness, and swelling associated with osteoarthritis.

- **Functional Improvement**: Improved joint mobility and physical function have been reported with MSM use.

Exercise Recovery and Muscle Pain

- **Reduction of Muscle Damage**: MSM may decrease markers of muscle damage following strenuous exercise.

- **Alleviation of Delayed Onset Muscle Soreness (DOMS)**: Supplementation can lessen the severity and duration of DOMS.

Skin Health

- **Dermatological Benefits**: MSM may improve skin hydration, elasticity, and reduce signs of aging by supporting collagen and keratin production.

- **Wound Healing**: Enhanced antioxidant capacity and anti-inflammatory effects may accelerate the healing of minor cuts and abrasions.

Allergies and Immune Modulation

- **Allergic Rhinitis Relief**: MSM may alleviate symptoms of seasonal allergies by reducing inflammatory mediators.

- **Immune System Support**: Modulation of immune cell activity can contribute to a balanced immune response.

Formulation Strategies

Oral Administration

- **Capsules and Tablets**: MSM is widely available in standardized doses ranging from 500 mg to 1500 mg per capsule or tablet.

- **Powder Form**: Offers flexibility in dosing and can be mixed with liquids; purity and solubility are important considerations.

Topical Applications with DMSO

- **Transdermal Delivery**: Combining MSM with DMSO in creams or gels can enhance skin penetration and localized effects.

- **Concentration Ratios**: Typical formulations may use MSM concentrations of 5% to 20% and DMSO concentrations of 25% to 50%.

Synergistic Formulations

- **Combination Products**: Some preparations include additional ingredients like glucosamine, chondroitin, or herbal extracts to support joint health.

- **Stability and Compatibility**: Formulations must ensure chemical stability and prevent degradation of active ingredients.

Safety and Tolerability

Adverse Effects

- **Gastrointestinal Symptoms**: Oral MSM is generally well-tolerated but may cause mild side effects like bloating, nausea, or diarrhea in some individuals.

- **Skin Reactions**: Topical use with DMSO may result in redness, itching, or burning sensations, particularly in sensitive individuals.

Toxicity Profile

- **Low Toxicity**: MSM has a high safety margin with low acute and chronic toxicity reported in animal studies.

- **Maximum Safe Dosage**: Clinical trials have used doses up to 6 grams per day without serious adverse effects.

Drug Interactions

- **Anticoagulant Medications**: Caution is advised when combining MSM with blood-thinning drugs due to potential additive effects.

- **DMSO Interaction**: DMSO may alter the absorption and metabolism of concomitant medications; consultation with a healthcare provider is recommended.

Contraindications

- **Pregnancy and Lactation**: Insufficient data exist regarding safety; use should be avoided unless prescribed by a physician.

- **Allergy to Sulfur Compounds**: Individuals with known allergies should exercise caution, although MSM allergies are rare.

Colloidal Silver

Introduction

Colloidal silver consists of microscopic silver particles suspended in a liquid medium, typically water. Historically used for its purported antimicrobial properties, colloidal silver has been marketed for various therapeutic applications, ranging from infection control to immune system support. This section examines the scientific evidence regarding colloidal silver, its potential interactions with dimethyl sulfoxide (DMSO), and the safety considerations associated with their combined use.

Chemical and Physical Properties of Colloidal Silver

Composition and Particle Size

- **Particle Characteristics**: Colloidal silver solutions contain silver nanoparticles varying in size from 1 to 100 nanometers. The particle size influences the colloidal stability, bioavailability, and biological activity of the silver particles.

- **Concentration**: Typically expressed in parts per million (ppm), concentrations can range from 5 ppm to over 500 ppm. Higher concentrations may increase the risk of adverse effects without corresponding therapeutic benefits.

Mechanisms of Action

- **Antimicrobial Activity**: Silver ions (Ag^+) released from the nanoparticles can interact with microbial cell membranes, proteins, and DNA, leading to cell death. The exact mechanisms involve disruption of electron transport systems, interference with essential enzymatic functions, and generation of reactive oxygen species (ROS).

- **Limitations**: The efficacy of colloidal silver as an antimicrobial agent in vivo remains poorly defined, with limited clinical evidence supporting its use.

Potential Therapeutic Applications

Antimicrobial Uses

- **Topical Application**: Silver-containing compounds have been used in wound dressings and topical creams to prevent or treat infections. However, these formulations typically involve silver sulfadiazine or other silver salts, not colloidal silver.

- **Systemic Use**: Oral ingestion or intravenous administration of colloidal silver for systemic infections lacks robust scientific support and poses significant safety concerns.

Alternative Medicine Claims

- **Immune Support**: Some proponents claim colloidal silver enhances immune function, though no credible scientific studies substantiate these assertions.

- **Chronic Conditions**: Colloidal silver has been marketed for conditions such as Lyme disease, chronic fatigue syndrome, and even cancer, but these uses are not supported by clinical evidence and are not recognized by medical authorities.

Interactions Between DMSO and Colloidal Silver

Solvent and Carrier Properties of DMSO

- **Enhanced Permeation**: DMSO's ability to increase skin permeability raises concerns that it may facilitate deeper penetration of silver particles into tissues when used concurrently.

- **Potential for Increased Absorption**: Combining DMSO with colloidal silver could theoretically enhance systemic absorption of silver, potentially leading to higher blood levels and increased risk of toxicity.

Chemical Compatibility

- **Stability Considerations**: Silver nanoparticles may aggregate or undergo oxidation when mixed with DMSO, potentially altering their size distribution and biological activity.

- **Chemical Reactions**: DMSO can act as a mild reducing agent, which might affect the oxidation state of silver particles. The implications of such reactions on safety and efficacy are not well-understood.

Safety and Toxicity

Risks of Silver Accumulation

- **Argyria**: Prolonged exposure to silver can lead to argyria, a condition characterized by irreversible bluish-gray discoloration of the skin, eyes, and mucous membranes due to silver deposition.

- **Organ Deposition**: Silver can accumulate in internal organs, including the liver, spleen, kidneys, and nervous system, potentially leading to functional impairments.

Cytotoxicity and Genotoxicity

- **Cellular Toxicity**: High concentrations of silver nanoparticles can induce cytotoxic effects, including oxidative stress, mitochondrial dysfunction, and apoptosis in human cells.

- **DNA Damage**: Some studies have reported genotoxic effects of silver nanoparticles, raising concerns about potential carcinogenicity with long-term exposure.

Allergic Reactions

- **Hypersensitivity**: Silver can elicit allergic contact dermatitis in susceptible individuals, presenting as skin rash, itching, and inflammation.

Regulatory Warnings

- **FDA Position**: The U.S. Food and Drug Administration (FDA) has issued warnings against the use of colloidal silver products marketed for medical purposes, citing a lack of evidence for safety and efficacy.

- **Health Canada and EMA**: Similar advisories have been issued by other regulatory agencies globally, discouraging the use of colloidal silver for therapeutic applications.

Clinical Evidence and Research Findings

Limited Efficacy Data

- **Inadequate Clinical Trials**: Few well-designed clinical trials have evaluated the therapeutic benefits of colloidal silver in humans. Existing studies often suffer from methodological flaws, small sample sizes, and lack of reproducibility.

- **Antimicrobial Claims**: While in vitro studies demonstrate antimicrobial activity of silver nanoparticles, translating these findings to clinical efficacy remains unproven.

Safety Concerns in Research

- **Adverse Events**: Case reports have documented argyria and other adverse effects in individuals using colloidal silver products, highlighting safety risks without corresponding therapeutic gains.

- **Dose-Response Relationship**: The lack of established dosing guidelines complicates the assessment of risk versus benefit, particularly when combined with penetration enhancers like DMSO.

Cannabis Extracts

Introduction

Cannabis extracts, derived from the *Cannabis sativa* plant, contain a variety of biologically active compounds known as cannabinoids, terpenes, and flavonoids. The most studied cannabinoids are delta-9-tetrahydrocannabinol (Δ^9-THC), responsible for the psychoactive effects, and cannabidiol (CBD), noted for its potential therapeutic properties without intoxicating effects. Combining dimethyl sulfoxide (DMSO) with cannabis extracts may enhance the transdermal delivery and efficacy of these bioactive compounds. This section explores the scientific rationale, potential therapeutic applications, formulation considerations, and safety aspects of using DMSO in conjunction with cannabis extracts.

Mechanisms of Interaction

DMSO as a Penetration Enhancer

- **Transdermal Absorption**: DMSO facilitates the permeation of compounds across the skin barrier by disrupting the stratum corneum lipid structure and altering protein conformation, thereby increasing membrane fluidity.

- **Solvent Properties**: DMSO's ability to dissolve both hydrophilic and lipophilic substances allows it to act as an effective carrier for the diverse range of compounds present in cannabis extracts.

Cannabinoid Bioavailability

- **Limited Oral Bioavailability**: Cannabinoids like THC and CBD have poor oral bioavailability due to first-pass hepatic metabolism and low water solubility.

- **Enhanced Delivery**: Utilizing DMSO may bypass gastrointestinal degradation and first-pass metabolism, potentially increasing systemic availability through transdermal administration.

Therapeutic Applications

Pain Management

- **Analgesic Effects**: Both THC and CBD exhibit analgesic properties through interaction with the endocannabinoid system, modulating pain signaling pathways.

- **Synergistic Action**: The combination with DMSO may enhance the delivery of cannabinoids to local tissues and systemic circulation, potentially improving pain relief in conditions such as neuropathic pain, arthritis, and musculoskeletal disorders.

Anti-Inflammatory Effects

- **Cannabinoid Activity**: CBD, in particular, has demonstrated anti-inflammatory effects by inhibiting pro-inflammatory cytokines and reducing oxidative stress.

- **Potential Enhancement**: DMSO may amplify these effects by increasing cannabinoid concentration at the site of inflammation and facilitating deeper tissue penetration.

Neurological Disorders

- **Neuroprotective Properties**: Cannabinoids have been studied for their potential in treating neurological conditions like multiple sclerosis, epilepsy, and Parkinson's disease.

- **Transdermal Delivery Advantages**: DMSO-assisted transdermal delivery may provide a steady release of cannabinoids, maintaining therapeutic plasma levels without the peaks and troughs associated with oral dosing.

Dermatological Conditions

- **Skin Disorders**: Topical application of cannabinoids has shown promise in treating conditions like psoriasis, eczema, and dermatitis due to their anti-inflammatory and anti-proliferative effects.

- **Enhanced Skin Absorption**: DMSO may improve the penetration of cannabinoids into the dermal layers, potentially increasing therapeutic efficacy.

Formulation Strategies

Selection of Cannabis Extracts

- **Full-Spectrum vs. Isolates**: Full-spectrum extracts contain a range of cannabinoids, terpenes, and flavonoids, which may exert an "entourage effect," enhancing therapeutic outcomes. Isolates contain a single cannabinoid, such as pure CBD.

- **Purity and Quality**: High-quality, contaminant-free extracts are essential to ensure safety and efficacy, especially when used transdermally with a penetration enhancer like DMSO.

Concentration Optimization

- **Cannabinoid Concentration**: Determining the optimal concentration of cannabinoids is crucial to achieve therapeutic effects while minimizing side effects.
- **DMSO Concentration**: Typically used at concentrations of 10% to 50% for transdermal formulations. Higher concentrations increase permeability but may also elevate the risk of skin irritation.

Formulation Types

- **Gels and Creams**: Incorporating DMSO and cannabis extracts into gels or creams can facilitate application and absorption.
- **Transdermal Patches**: Controlled-release patches may offer sustained delivery of cannabinoids, potentially enhancing compliance and therapeutic outcomes.

Safety and Toxicity

Skin Irritation

- **DMSO Effects**: DMSO can cause skin redness, itching, and burning sensations, particularly at higher concentrations.
- **Cannabinoid Effects**: Generally well-tolerated topically, but some individuals may experience allergic reactions or dermatitis.

Systemic Absorption Risks

- **Psychoactive Effects**: Enhanced transdermal absorption of THC could lead to systemic psychoactive effects, such as euphoria, dizziness, or anxiety.
- **Dose Control**: Precise dosing is essential to avoid unintentional intoxication, especially with full-spectrum extracts containing THC.

Drug Interactions

- **Metabolic Enzymes**: Cannabinoids can inhibit cytochrome P450 enzymes, potentially affecting the metabolism of other medications.
- **Combined Effects**: DMSO may alter drug absorption and metabolism, necessitating careful monitoring when patients are on concurrent medications.

Practical Application Guidelines

Medical Supervision

- **Healthcare Involvement**: Use should be supervised by a healthcare professional knowledgeable in cannabinoid therapy and DMSO applications.
- **Patient Monitoring**: Regular assessment for efficacy and adverse effects is essential.

Application Techniques

- **Skin Preparation**: Clean the application area thoroughly to reduce the risk of contamination and unintended absorption of impurities.
- **Administration**: Apply a measured dose using appropriate applicators, avoiding mucous membranes and broken skin unless directed by a physician.

Dosage Recommendations

- **Individualized Dosing**: Start with the lowest effective dose, gradually adjusting based on therapeutic response and tolerance.
- **Frequency**: Follow a consistent dosing schedule as advised by a healthcare provider.

Chapter 4: DMSO for Specific Ailments

Pain Management

Introduction

Pain management is a critical component of medical care, aiming to alleviate discomfort and improve the quality of life for individuals suffering from acute or chronic pain conditions. Dimethyl sulfoxide (DMSO) has attracted scientific interest for its potential analgesic and anti-inflammatory properties. This section explores the mechanisms by which DMSO may contribute to pain relief, examines clinical applications, reviews current research findings, and discusses safety considerations.

Mechanisms of Action in Pain Relief

Anti-Inflammatory Effects

- **Cytokine Modulation**: DMSO has been shown to inhibit the production of pro-inflammatory cytokines such as interleukin-6 (IL-6) and tumor necrosis factor-alpha (TNF-α). By reducing these mediators, DMSO may decrease inflammation and associated pain.

- **Inhibition of Prostaglandin Synthesis**: DMSO interferes with the cyclooxygenase (COX) pathway, leading to decreased production of prostaglandins, which are lipid compounds that sensitize nociceptors and enhance pain perception.

Antioxidant Properties

- **Reactive Oxygen Species Scavenging**: DMSO acts as a free radical scavenger, neutralizing reactive oxygen species (ROS) that contribute to cellular damage and inflammation. This antioxidant activity may protect tissues and reduce pain caused by oxidative stress.

Modulation of Nerve Conduction

- **Alteration of Membrane Permeability**: DMSO can influence the permeability of neuronal cell membranes, potentially affecting the transmission of pain signals.

- **Ion Channel Interaction**: It may modulate ion channels involved in nerve excitation, such as sodium and calcium channels, leading to decreased neuronal excitability and pain signaling.

Clinical Applications in Pain Management

Musculoskeletal Pain

- **Osteoarthritis**: Topical DMSO has been investigated for reducing joint pain and improving function in osteoarthritis patients. Some studies report modest pain relief and enhanced mobility.

- **Rheumatoid Arthritis**: Due to its anti-inflammatory properties, DMSO may alleviate joint inflammation and pain in rheumatoid arthritis, although more robust clinical evidence is needed.

- **Tendinopathies**: DMSO's ability to penetrate deep tissues makes it a candidate for treating tendon-related pain by delivering anti-inflammatory effects directly to the affected area.

Neuropathic Pain

- **Peripheral Neuropathy**: DMSO may offer relief in conditions involving nerve damage by reducing inflammation around nerves and modulating pain signal transmission.

- **Complex Regional Pain Syndrome (CRPS)**: Some case studies suggest that topical DMSO can alleviate pain and other symptoms associated with CRPS, possibly due to its anti-inflammatory and antioxidant effects.

Postoperative Pain

- **Surgical Recovery**: DMSO has been explored as an adjunct therapy to reduce pain and inflammation following surgical procedures, potentially speeding up recovery times.

Administration Methods

Topical Application

- **Gels and Creams**: DMSO is most commonly applied topically in gel or cream formulations, allowing direct action on affected areas with minimal systemic absorption.

- **Application Protocol**: Concentrations of 50–70% DMSO are typically used for pain management. The area should be clean, and application should follow guidelines to maximize efficacy and minimize skin irritation.

Combination Therapies

- **With Other Analgesics**: DMSO may be combined with other topical pain relievers, such as nonsteroidal anti-inflammatory drugs (NSAIDs), to enhance their absorption and effectiveness.

- **Transdermal Delivery Systems**: Research is exploring the use of DMSO in transdermal patches to provide controlled release of analgesic agents for sustained pain relief.

Safety and Side Effects

Local Adverse Effects

- **Skin Irritation**: Common side effects include redness, itching, and a burning sensation at the application site. These are generally mild and resolve upon discontinuation.

- **Dermatitis**: Prolonged use or high concentrations may lead to dermatitis or blistering in sensitive individuals.

Systemic Effects

- **Breath and Body Odor**: DMSO can cause a garlic-like odor due to its metabolism to dimethyl sulfide, which may be socially undesirable but is harmless.

- **Allergic Reactions**: Although rare, hypersensitivity reactions can occur, manifesting as hives, swelling, or difficulty breathing, requiring immediate medical attention.

Drug Interactions

- **Enhanced Absorption**: DMSO's ability to increase skin permeability may lead to higher systemic levels of concurrently applied medications, necessitating caution to avoid toxicity.

- **Contraindications**: Patients using certain medications or with specific medical conditions should consult a healthcare professional before using DMSO.

Guidelines for Use

Patient Assessment

- **Medical History Review**: Evaluate for potential contraindications, such as allergies, liver or kidney impairment, and concurrent medication use.

- **Skin Examination**: Assess the application area for open wounds or dermatological conditions that may increase absorption or risk of irritation.

Application Recommendations

- **Concentration Selection**: Start with lower concentrations to assess tolerance, especially in patients with sensitive skin.

- **Frequency**: Apply DMSO two to three times daily or as directed by a healthcare provider, avoiding excessive use.

- **Hygiene Practices**: Ensure the skin is clean before application to prevent the absorption of contaminants.

Introduction

Arthritis encompasses a group of conditions characterized by inflammation of the joints, leading to pain, stiffness, and decreased mobility. The most common forms are osteoarthritis (OA), resulting from cartilage degeneration, and rheumatoid arthritis (RA), an autoimmune disorder targeting joint linings. Joint pain associated with arthritis significantly impacts the quality of life and functional capacity of affected individuals. Dimethyl sulfoxide (DMSO) has been investigated for its potential therapeutic effects in managing arthritis and joint pain due to its unique physicochemical properties and biological activities. This section delves into the scientific evidence supporting the use of DMSO in arthritis treatment, elucidates its mechanisms of action, examines clinical study findings, and discusses practical considerations for its application.

Pathophysiology of Arthritis

Osteoarthritis (OA)

- **Cartilage Degradation**: OA is characterized by the progressive breakdown of articular cartilage, leading to bone-on-bone contact, pain, and joint deformity.

- **Inflammatory Mediators**: While traditionally considered a degenerative disease, low-grade inflammation involving cytokines like interleukin-1β (IL-1β) and tumor necrosis factor-alpha (TNF-α) contributes to cartilage degradation and pain in OA.

- **Mechanical Stress**: Joint overuse, obesity, and mechanical injuries accelerate cartilage wear and osteophyte formation.

Rheumatoid Arthritis (RA)

- **Autoimmune Response**: RA involves an aberrant immune attack on synovial membranes, resulting in chronic inflammation, synovial hyperplasia, and joint destruction.

- **Cytokine Cascade**: Pro-inflammatory cytokines such as TNF-α, IL-6, and IL-17 play pivotal roles in perpetuating inflammation and joint damage.

- **Systemic Effects**: RA can affect multiple organ systems, causing systemic symptoms like fatigue and anemia.

Mechanisms of DMSO in Arthritis Management

Anti-Inflammatory Actions

- **Cytokine Suppression**: DMSO inhibits the production and activity of pro-inflammatory cytokines, reducing synovial inflammation and cartilage degradation.

- **Modulation of Immune Cells**: It affects the function of macrophages and lymphocytes, attenuating the autoimmune responses in RA.

- **Inhibition of Metalloproteinases**: DMSO may suppress matrix metalloproteinases (MMPs), enzymes that degrade cartilage extracellular matrix components.

Antioxidant Properties

- **Free Radical Scavenging**: By neutralizing ROS, DMSO protects chondrocytes (cartilage cells) from oxidative damage, which contributes to disease progression.

- **Lipid Peroxidation Prevention**: It inhibits lipid peroxidation in cell membranes, preserving cellular integrity in joint tissues.

Analgesic Effects

- **Nociceptor Modulation**: DMSO may reduce the sensitivity of pain receptors in joints, alleviating discomfort associated with arthritis.

- **Neural Transmission Alteration**: It can interfere with the transmission of pain signals by modulating ion channels and neurotransmitter release.

Penetration Enhancement

- **Transdermal Delivery**: DMSO's ability to penetrate the skin allows it to deliver therapeutic agents directly to the affected joints when used in combination with other medications.

Administration Methods Specific to Arthritis

Topical Application

- **Concentration**: DMSO concentrations ranging from 50% to 70% are commonly used for arthritis treatment.

- **Formulations**: Available as gels, creams, or solutions, sometimes combined with other anti-inflammatory agents.

- **Application Site**: Applied directly over the affected joints, ensuring clean skin to optimize absorption and reduce contamination risks.

- **Frequency**: Typically administered two to three times daily, as advised by a healthcare professional.

Combination Therapies

- **With NSAIDs**: DMSO can enhance the transdermal delivery of NSAIDs like diclofenac, potentially increasing their local effectiveness.

- **With Corticosteroids**: Combining DMSO with topical corticosteroids may provide synergistic anti-inflammatory effects.

- **Natural Compounds**: Incorporation of substances like MSM (methylsulfonylmethane) or glucosamine may support joint health when used with DMSO.

Safety Considerations

Skin Reactions

- **Irritation Potential**: Higher concentrations of DMSO may cause skin irritation, redness, or itching.

- **Hypersensitivity Testing**: A patch test is recommended before initiating treatment to assess individual tolerance.

Systemic Absorption Risks

- **Contaminant Absorption**: DMSO's penetration-enhancing properties necessitate careful skin cleaning to prevent unintended absorption of harmful substances.

- **Medication Interactions**: Enhanced absorption of co-administered drugs may alter their systemic levels, requiring dosage adjustments.

Contraindications

- **Medical Conditions**: Patients with liver or kidney impairments should use DMSO cautiously due to altered metabolism and excretion.

- **Pregnancy and Lactation**: The safety of DMSO during pregnancy or breastfeeding is not well-established; its use is generally discouraged in these populations.

Tendonitis and Muscle Pain

Introduction

Tendonitis and muscle pain are prevalent musculoskeletal conditions that can significantly impair mobility and quality of life. Tendonitis refers to the inflammation of tendons, the fibrous connective tissues that attach muscles to bones, often resulting from overuse or acute injury. Muscle pain, or myalgia, can arise from strains, sprains, or systemic conditions affecting muscle tissue. Dimethyl sulfoxide (DMSO) has garnered attention for its potential therapeutic effects in alleviating these conditions due to its anti-inflammatory, analgesic, and membrane-penetrating properties. This section examines the scientific basis for using DMSO in treating tendonitis and muscle pain, explores clinical evidence, and discusses practical considerations for its application.

Pathophysiology of Tendonitis and Muscle Pain

Tendonitis

- **Inflammatory Response**: Tendonitis involves an acute or chronic inflammatory process characterized by the infiltration of inflammatory cells, increased production of cytokines, and local edema within the tendon sheath.

- **Degenerative Changes**: Prolonged inflammation can lead to tendinosis, a degeneration of the tendon fibers marked by collagen disorganization and microtears.

- **Mechanical Overload**: Repetitive stress, improper biomechanics, or sudden increases in physical activity can precipitate tendon injury and inflammation.

Muscle Pain

- **Muscle Strain**: Overstretching or tearing of muscle fibers due to excessive force can cause acute pain and inflammation.

- **Delayed Onset Muscle Soreness (DOMS)**: Microtrauma from unaccustomed or intense exercise leads to muscle soreness peaking 24–72 hours post-activity.

- **Myofascial Pain Syndrome**: Trigger points within muscle tissue can cause localized pain and referred pain patterns.

Mechanisms of DMSO in Treating Tendonitis and Muscle Pain

Anti-Inflammatory Effects

- **Cytokine Modulation**: DMSO inhibits the synthesis and release of pro-inflammatory cytokines such as interleukin-1 beta (IL-1β) and tumor necrosis factor-alpha (TNF-α), reducing inflammatory cascades in tendon and muscle tissues.

- **Leukocyte Inhibition**: It suppresses the migration and activation of neutrophils and macrophages at sites of injury, decreasing tissue damage from inflammatory mediators.

Analgesic Properties

- **Nociceptor Desensitization**: DMSO can modulate the activity of peripheral nociceptors, diminishing pain signal transmission from affected areas.

- **Neural Membrane Stabilization**: By affecting ion channel permeability, DMSO may stabilize neuronal membranes, reducing hyperexcitability associated with pain.

Enhanced Membrane Penetration

- **Transdermal Absorption**: DMSO's ability to penetrate biological membranes facilitates the delivery of therapeutic agents directly to inflamed tendons and muscles.

- **Increased Bioavailability**: It enhances the local concentration of co-administered medications, potentially improving their therapeutic efficacy.

Antioxidant Activity

- **Free Radical Scavenging**: DMSO neutralizes reactive oxygen species (ROS), mitigating oxidative stress that contributes to tissue inflammation and pain.

- **Lipid Peroxidation Inhibition**: It protects cell membranes from lipid peroxidation, preserving cellular integrity in muscle and tendon fibers.

Clinical Evidence

Tendonitis Treatment

- **Lateral Epicondylitis (Tennis Elbow)**:

- o *Study Findings*: Topical application of DMSO has been associated with reduced pain and improved grip strength in patients with lateral epicondylitis.

- o *Mechanism*: The anti-inflammatory and analgesic effects may alleviate tendon inflammation and associated symptoms.

- **Achilles Tendonitis**:

  - o *Clinical Reports*: Patients using DMSO experienced decreased swelling and pain, facilitating a return to normal activities.

  - o *Combination Therapy*: DMSO combined with physical therapy showed enhanced recovery compared to physical therapy alone.

Muscle Pain Management

- **Acute Muscle Strains**:

  - o *Pain Reduction*: Application of DMSO shortly after injury has been reported to decrease pain intensity and muscle stiffness.

  - o *Functional Improvement*: Accelerated recovery times and improved range of motion have been observed in some cases.

- **Delayed Onset Muscle Soreness (DOMS)**:

  - o *Exercise Recovery*: Athletes using DMSO reported less severe muscle soreness and quicker recovery post-exercise.

  - o *Inflammation Markers*: Reductions in creatine kinase levels, a marker of muscle damage, were noted in some studies.

Limitations and Considerations

- **Variability in Results**: Inconsistent outcomes across studies highlight the need for standardized research protocols.

- **Sample Size Constraints**: Many studies involve small cohorts, limiting statistical significance.

- **Placebo Effects**: The subjective nature of pain necessitates rigorous placebo-controlled trials to validate findings.

Administration Methods

Topical Application

- **Concentration Selection**:

  - o *Tendonitis*: DMSO concentrations of 50% to 70% are commonly used for tendon inflammation.

  - o *Muscle Pain*: Concentrations may range from 25% to 50%, balancing efficacy with skin tolerability.

- **Application Protocol**:

  - o *Skin Preparation*: Cleanse the area with mild soap and water to remove oils and contaminants.

  - o *Dosage and Frequency*: Apply a thin layer to the affected area two to three times daily or as directed by a healthcare professional.

  - o *Massage Technique*: Gentle massage may enhance absorption but should be performed carefully to avoid aggravating the injury.

Combination Therapies

- **Nonsteroidal Anti-Inflammatory Drugs (NSAIDs)**:

  - o *Synergistic Effect*: DMSO can enhance the transdermal delivery of NSAIDs like ibuprofen or diclofenac, potentially increasing their anti-inflammatory action.

- **Local Anesthetics**:

    o *Pain Relief*: Combining DMSO with lidocaine may provide immediate analgesia for severe pain episodes.

- **Herbal Extracts**:

    o *Adjunctive Use*: Natural anti-inflammatory agents like arnica or menthol may be included in formulations, although clinical evidence is limited.

Safety and Side Effects

Local Adverse Effects

- **Skin Irritation**: Redness, itching, and a burning sensation may occur, particularly with higher concentrations.

- **Dermatitis**: Prolonged use or sensitivity may lead to contact dermatitis; discontinuation typically resolves symptoms.

Systemic Considerations

- **Odor and Taste Alterations**: A garlic-like odor on the breath and skin is common due to DMSO metabolism to dimethyl sulfide.

- **Allergic Reactions**: Rare cases of hypersensitivity reactions necessitate immediate medical attention.

Precautions

- **Drug Interactions**: Enhanced absorption of other medications may increase systemic levels, requiring monitoring and possible dosage adjustments.

- **Contraindications**:

    o *Pregnancy and Lactation*: Use is not recommended due to insufficient safety data.

    o *Renal or Hepatic Impairment*: Caution is advised as DMSO is metabolized in the liver and excreted by the kidneys.

Practical Application Guidelines

Patient Assessment

- **Medical History Review**: Evaluate for allergies, existing medical conditions, and concurrent medication use.

- **Injury Evaluation**: Confirm the diagnosis and severity of tendon or muscle injury to determine the appropriateness of DMSO therapy.

Application Instructions

- **Dosage Adherence**: Follow prescribed concentrations and application frequency to minimize side effects.

- **Hygiene Measures**: Ensure hands and application sites are clean to prevent contamination and unintended absorption of substances.

- **Protective Measures**: Use gloves when applying DMSO to prevent personal exposure and reduce odor transfer.

Monitoring and Follow-Up

- **Symptom Tracking**: Document pain levels, functional improvements, and any adverse reactions.

- **Treatment Adjustment**: Modify concentration or frequency based on patient response and tolerance.

- **Rehabilitation Integration**: Incorporate DMSO therapy within a broader treatment plan, including rest, physical therapy, and gradual return to activity.

Introduction

Nerve pain, or neuropathic pain, arises from damage or dysfunction within the nervous system, leading to chronic and often debilitating sensations such as burning, tingling, or electric shocks. Neuropathy encompasses a range of conditions affecting peripheral nerves, including diabetic neuropathy, post-herpetic neuralgia, and chemotherapy-induced neuropathy. Traditional pain management strategies often provide limited relief for neuropathic pain, prompting interest in alternative therapies. Dimethyl sulfoxide (DMSO) has been investigated for its potential role in alleviating nerve pain due to its unique pharmacological properties. This section explores the scientific basis for DMSO's use in neuropathy, reviews clinical evidence, and discusses practical considerations for its application.

Pathophysiology of Neuropathic Pain

Mechanisms of Nerve Damage

- **Peripheral Nerve Injury**: Physical trauma, metabolic disorders, infections, or exposure to neurotoxic agents can damage peripheral nerves, disrupting normal signal transmission.

- **Demyelination**: Loss of the myelin sheath, which insulates nerve fibers, leads to aberrant electrical conduction and heightened pain sensitivity.

- **Axonal Degeneration**: Damage to the axon impairs nerve function and can result in neuronal death.

Altered Pain Signaling

- **Ectopic Discharge**: Damaged nerves may generate spontaneous electrical impulses, leading to persistent pain sensations without external stimuli.

- **Central Sensitization**: Prolonged nociceptive input can sensitize neurons in the dorsal horn of the spinal cord, amplifying pain signals.

- **Inflammatory Mediators**: Release of cytokines, chemokines, and growth factors contributes to nerve inflammation and pain hypersensitivity.

Mechanisms of DMSO in Neuropathic Pain Management

Anti-Inflammatory Actions

- **Cytokine Inhibition**: DMSO suppresses pro-inflammatory cytokines such as interleukin-1 beta (IL-1β) and tumor necrosis factor-alpha (TNF-α), which play a role in neuroinflammation.

- **Reduction of Neuroinflammation**: By decreasing the infiltration of inflammatory cells and mediators at sites of nerve injury, DMSO may alleviate inflammation-induced nerve pain.

Neuroprotective Effects

- **Free Radical Scavenging**: DMSO's antioxidant properties enable it to neutralize reactive oxygen species (ROS), reducing oxidative stress that contributes to neuronal damage.

- **Membrane Stabilization**: It may protect neuronal cell membranes from lipid peroxidation, preserving nerve integrity.

Modulation of Ion Channels

- **Sodium and Calcium Channels**: DMSO can influence ion channel function, potentially reducing neuronal hyperexcitability associated with neuropathic pain.

- **Inhibition of Ectopic Discharges**: By stabilizing ion fluxes, DMSO may decrease spontaneous nerve firing that leads to pain.

Enhanced Drug Delivery

- **Transdermal Penetration**: DMSO enhances the absorption of co-administered analgesic agents, potentially improving their efficacy in targeting nerve pain.

- **Blood-Brain Barrier Permeability**: It may facilitate the delivery of therapeutic compounds across the blood-brain barrier, affecting central pain pathways.

Administration Methods Specific to Neuropathic Pain

Topical Application

- **Concentration Selection**: DMSO concentrations of 50% are commonly used for neuropathic pain, balancing efficacy with skin tolerability.

- **Application Site**: Applied directly over the areas of nerve pain, ensuring the skin is intact and free from wounds.

- **Frequency**: Typically administered two to three times daily, as recommended by a healthcare professional.

- **Adjunctive Agents**: May be combined with other topical analgesics like lidocaine or menthol to enhance pain relief.

Oral Administration

- **Limited Use**: Oral ingestion of DMSO is not widely recommended due to insufficient evidence of efficacy and potential side effects.

- **Clinical Caution**: Any consideration of oral DMSO should be under strict medical supervision within a research setting.

Combination with Systemic Therapies

- **Enhanced Drug Delivery**: DMSO may improve the efficacy of systemic neuropathic pain medications by facilitating their transport across biological barriers.

- **Monitoring Required**: Close monitoring is essential to avoid increased systemic exposure leading to toxicity.

Safety and Side Effects

Local Adverse Effects

- **Skin Irritation**: Possible redness, itching, or burning at the application site; performing a patch test can help assess sensitivity.

- **Dermatitis Risk**: Prolonged use may lead to contact dermatitis in susceptible individuals.

Systemic Effects

- **Odor**: The metabolism of DMSO to dimethyl sulfide may result in a transient garlic-like odor on breath and skin.

- **Allergic Reactions**: Rare but may include hives, swelling, or difficulty breathing, requiring immediate medical attention.

Drug Interactions

- **Enhanced Absorption**: DMSO can increase the systemic absorption of other medications, potentially altering their effects.

- **Contraindications**: Patients taking multiple medications should consult a healthcare provider to assess interaction risks.

Precautions

- **Pregnancy and Lactation**: The safety of DMSO during pregnancy or breastfeeding is not established; use is generally discouraged.

- **Pre-existing Conditions**: Caution in patients with liver, kidney, or cardiovascular conditions due to altered metabolism and excretion.

Practical Considerations for Clinical Use

Patient Assessment

- **Comprehensive Evaluation**: Assess the underlying cause of neuropathic pain to determine if DMSO is an appropriate adjunct therapy.

- **Medical History**: Review for potential allergies, contraindications, and concurrent medication use.

Application Guidelines

- **Skin Preparation**: Clean the area thoroughly to prevent absorption of contaminants.

- **Dosage Adherence**: Follow prescribed concentrations and application frequencies.

- **Protective Measures**: Use gloves during application to avoid self-exposure.

Monitoring and Follow-Up

- **Efficacy Assessment**: Regularly evaluate pain levels, functional improvements, and quality of life measures.

- **Side Effect Surveillance**: Monitor for adverse reactions, adjusting treatment as necessary.

- **Patient Education**: Instruct on proper application techniques, storage, and handling of DMSO.

Inflammation Reduction

Introduction

Inflammation is a complex biological response to harmful stimuli such as pathogens, damaged cells, or irritants. It is a protective mechanism intended to eliminate the initial cause of cell injury, clear out necrotic cells and tissues, and establish repair. However, chronic inflammation can lead to a range of diseases, including autoimmune disorders, cardiovascular diseases, and neurodegenerative conditions. Dimethyl sulfoxide (DMSO) has been studied for its anti-inflammatory properties, which may offer therapeutic benefits in managing various inflammatory conditions. This section explores the mechanisms by which DMSO reduces inflammation, examines clinical applications beyond pain management, reviews scientific evidence, and discusses safety considerations.

Mechanisms of Anti-Inflammatory Action

Modulation of Cytokine Production

- **Inhibition of Pro-Inflammatory Cytokines**: DMSO has been shown to suppress the production of key pro-inflammatory cytokines such as interleukin-1 beta (IL-1β), interleukin-6 (IL-6), and tumor necrosis factor-alpha (TNF-α). By downregulating these cytokines, DMSO can attenuate the inflammatory response at the molecular level.

- **Enhancement of Anti-Inflammatory Cytokines**: It may promote the expression of anti-inflammatory cytokines like interleukin-10 (IL-10), contributing to a shift towards an anti-inflammatory state.

Inhibition of Nuclear Factor Kappa B (NF-κB) Pathway

- **Transcription Factor Suppression**: DMSO can inhibit the activation of NF-κB, a critical transcription factor that regulates the expression of various inflammatory genes. By preventing NF-κB translocation to the nucleus, DMSO reduces the transcription of inflammatory mediators.

Reduction of Reactive Oxygen Species (ROS)

- **Antioxidant Activity**: DMSO acts as a scavenger of reactive oxygen species, which are generated during inflammation and contribute to tissue damage. By neutralizing ROS, DMSO mitigates oxidative stress and subsequent inflammatory signaling.

Inhibition of Inflammasome Activation

- **NLRP3 Inflammasome**: DMSO has been observed to inhibit the activation of the NLRP3 inflammasome, a multiprotein complex involved in the maturation of pro-inflammatory cytokines like IL-1β. This inhibition reduces the amplification of inflammatory responses.

Suppression of Adhesion Molecule Expression

- **Leukocyte Adhesion**: DMSO can decrease the expression of adhesion molecules such as intercellular adhesion molecule-1 (ICAM-1) on endothelial cells. This reduction limits the recruitment and infiltration of leukocytes into inflamed tissues.

Clinical Applications in Inflammatory Conditions

Autoimmune Diseases

- **Systemic Lupus Erythematosus (SLE)**: DMSO's immunomodulatory effects may benefit patients with SLE by reducing autoantibody production and inflammatory cytokine levels.

- **Multiple Sclerosis (MS)**: Preclinical studies suggest that DMSO might inhibit demyelination and neuroinflammation, potentially slowing disease progression in MS.

Inflammatory Bowel Disease (IBD)

- **Ulcerative Colitis and Crohn's Disease**: DMSO's anti-inflammatory and antioxidant properties could help reduce intestinal inflammation, mucosal damage, and oxidative stress associated with IBD.

Dermatological Inflammatory Conditions

- **Psoriasis**: Topical DMSO may alleviate psoriatic lesions by reducing keratinocyte proliferation and inflammation.

- **Atopic Dermatitis**: Its ability to modulate immune responses might help in managing eczema by decreasing skin inflammation and itching.

Respiratory Inflammation

- **Asthma and Chronic Obstructive Pulmonary Disease (COPD)**: DMSO may reduce airway inflammation and hyperresponsiveness by inhibiting inflammatory mediators in the respiratory tract.

Cardiovascular Inflammation

- **Atherosclerosis**: By suppressing endothelial inflammation and oxidative stress, DMSO might slow the progression of atherosclerotic plaque formation.

Scientific Evidence and Research Findings

Preclinical Studies

- **Animal Models**: In rodent models of autoimmune encephalomyelitis (a model for MS), DMSO administration reduced neurological deficits and inflammatory cell infiltration.

- **Cell Culture Studies**: DMSO inhibited the activation of macrophages and T cells, leading to decreased production of inflammatory cytokines and nitric oxide.

Clinical Studies

- **Inflammatory Skin Conditions**: Small clinical trials have demonstrated improvements in psoriasis severity scores with topical DMSO applications.

- **Gastrointestinal Inflammation**: Limited studies suggest that rectal administration of DMSO may reduce symptoms and inflammatory markers in ulcerative colitis patients.

Limitations of Current Research

- **Study Design**: Many studies are preliminary, with small sample sizes and lack of placebo controls.

- **Heterogeneity**: Variations in DMSO concentrations, administration routes, and treatment durations make it challenging to compare results across studies.

- **Need for Large-Scale Trials**: Comprehensive clinical trials are necessary to validate efficacy and establish standardized treatment protocols.

Administration Methods for Inflammation Reduction

Topical Application

- **Dermatological Conditions**: DMSO creams or gels at concentrations of 50% or lower are applied directly to affected skin areas.

- **Transdermal Delivery**: For systemic inflammatory conditions, DMSO may be used as a vehicle to deliver anti-inflammatory drugs through the skin.

Oral Administration

- **Systemic Effects**: Oral DMSO has been explored for systemic inflammation but is limited by potential side effects and lack of regulatory approval.

- **Gastrointestinal Targeting**: Enteric-coated formulations aim to deliver DMSO to the intestines, potentially benefiting IBD patients.

Intravesical Administration

- **Bladder Inflammation**: DMSO is FDA-approved for intravesical instillation in interstitial cystitis to reduce bladder inflammation and pain.

Inhalation Therapy

- **Respiratory Conditions**: Nebulized DMSO has been investigated for delivering anti-inflammatory effects directly to the airways in asthma and COPD, though safety concerns limit its use.

Safety and Side Effects

Local Reactions

- **Skin Irritation**: May cause redness, dryness, or itching when applied topically; usually mild and transient.

- **Mucous Membrane Sensitivity**: Oral or inhaled DMSO can irritate mucous membranes, leading to discomfort.

Systemic Effects

- **Breath and Body Odor**: A garlic-like smell is common due to dimethyl sulfide production during metabolism.

- **Gastrointestinal Symptoms**: Oral administration may cause nausea, diarrhea, or abdominal cramps.

Toxicity Concerns

- **Reproductive Effects**: Limited data suggest potential teratogenic effects; contraindicated in pregnancy.

- **Neurotoxicity**: High doses may lead to dizziness, headache, or sedation.

Drug Interactions

- **Medication Absorption**: DMSO may enhance the absorption of co-administered drugs, necessitating dosage adjustments.

- **Enzyme Modulation**: It can affect hepatic enzymes involved in drug metabolism, impacting the efficacy of other medications.

Practical Considerations

Patient Selection

- **Medical Evaluation**: Assess for contraindications such as liver or kidney impairment, pregnancy, or allergy to DMSO.

- **Tailored Therapy**: Customize concentration and administration route based on the specific inflammatory condition and patient tolerance.

Monitoring and Follow-Up

- **Effectiveness Assessment**: Regularly evaluate symptom improvement and inflammatory markers where applicable.

- **Side Effect Management**: Monitor for adverse reactions, adjusting treatment as necessary.

Regulatory Compliance

- **Approval Status**: DMSO is approved for certain indications; off-label use should be guided by clinical judgment and patient consent.

- **Quality Assurance**: Use pharmaceutical-grade DMSO to ensure purity and reduce the risk of contaminants.

Wound Healing

Introduction

Wound healing is a complex physiological process that restores the integrity of damaged tissues after injury. It involves a coordinated series of events, including hemostasis, inflammation, proliferation, and remodeling. Effective wound healing is essential for preventing infection, minimizing scarring, and restoring normal function. Despite advances in medical science, impaired wound healing remains a significant clinical challenge, particularly in chronic wounds associated with diabetes, vascular insufficiency, and immunodeficiency.

Dimethyl sulfoxide (DMSO) has been investigated for its potential to enhance wound healing due to its anti-inflammatory, antioxidant, and antimicrobial properties, as well as its ability to act as a penetration enhancer. This section explores the mechanisms by which DMSO may facilitate wound repair, examines relevant scientific studies, and discusses practical considerations for its clinical application.

Mechanisms of DMSO in Wound Healing

Anti-Inflammatory Effects

- **Modulation of Inflammatory Response**: DMSO can reduce excessive inflammation by inhibiting the production of pro-inflammatory cytokines such as interleukin-1 beta (IL-1β) and tumor necrosis factor-alpha (TNF-α). By attenuating the inflammatory phase, DMSO may prevent prolonged inflammation that can impede wound healing.

Antioxidant Properties

- **Scavenging Reactive Oxygen Species (ROS)**: DMSO acts as a free radical scavenger, neutralizing ROS that can cause cellular damage and delay healing. By reducing oxidative stress, DMSO supports the survival and function of cells critical for tissue repair.

Enhancement of Collagen Synthesis

- **Promotion of Fibroblast Activity**: DMSO may stimulate fibroblast proliferation and collagen production, essential for the formation of new extracellular matrix and granulation tissue during the proliferative phase of wound healing.

Angiogenesis Promotion

- **Stimulation of Neovascularization**: By encouraging the formation of new blood vessels, DMSO can improve oxygen and nutrient delivery to the wound site, facilitating tissue regeneration and remodeling.

Antimicrobial Effects

- **Inhibition of Microbial Growth**: DMSO possesses antimicrobial properties against a range of pathogens, including bacteria and fungi. Reducing microbial load at the wound site can prevent infection and associated complications.

Penetration Enhancement

- **Facilitation of Drug Delivery**: DMSO enhances the transdermal absorption of co-administered therapeutic agents, such as antibiotics and growth factors, potentially increasing their efficacy in wound management.

Scientific Evidence and Research Findings

Preclinical Studies

- **Animal Models**: In studies involving rodents with induced wounds, topical application of DMSO accelerated wound closure compared to control groups. Histological analysis revealed increased collagen deposition and angiogenesis in DMSO-treated wounds.

- **Cell Culture Studies**: In vitro experiments demonstrated that DMSO promotes fibroblast proliferation and enhances the expression of genes involved in extracellular matrix formation.

Clinical Studies

- **Burn Wounds**: Limited clinical trials have explored the use of DMSO in treating burn injuries. Patients receiving topical DMSO showed reduced pain, decreased inflammation, and faster epithelialization.

- **Chronic Ulcers**: Case reports suggest that DMSO may improve healing rates in chronic ulcers, such as diabetic foot ulcers and pressure sores, though robust clinical trials are lacking.

Limitations of Current Research

- **Small Sample Sizes**: Many studies have small participant numbers, limiting the ability to generalize findings.

- **Lack of Standardization**: Variability in DMSO concentrations, formulations, and application protocols makes it difficult to compare results across studies.

- **Need for Controlled Trials**: High-quality randomized controlled trials are necessary to establish the efficacy and safety of DMSO in wound healing conclusively.

Practical Applications in Wound Management

Topical Application

- **Formulations**: DMSO is applied as a gel, cream, or solution at concentrations typically ranging from 25% to 70%, depending on the type and severity of the wound.

- **Application Protocol**: The wound area should be cleaned thoroughly before applying DMSO to prevent the absorption of contaminants. DMSO is applied gently to the wound bed and surrounding skin, usually two to three times daily.

Combination Therapies

- **With Antimicrobials**: DMSO can be combined with topical antibiotics or antifungal agents to enhance their penetration and effectiveness against wound infections.

- **With Growth Factors**: Incorporating growth factors or cytokines into DMSO formulations may promote tissue regeneration and accelerate healing.

- **With Natural Compounds**: DMSO may be used alongside natural agents like honey or aloe vera, known for their wound-healing properties, though scientific evidence for such combinations is limited.

Safety and Side Effects

Local Reactions

- **Skin Irritation**: DMSO may cause redness, itching, or a burning sensation at the application site. These effects are generally mild and transient.

- **Delayed Wound Healing**: In some cases, improper use of DMSO, particularly at high concentrations, may delay healing or cause tissue maceration.

Systemic Effects

- **Odor**: A garlic-like odor on the breath and skin is common due to DMSO metabolism, which may be socially undesirable but is not harmful.

- **Allergic Reactions**: Rarely, individuals may experience hypersensitivity reactions to DMSO, necessitating discontinuation of use.

Precautions

- **Sterility**: Maintaining sterility is crucial when applying DMSO to open wounds to prevent infection.

- **Quality of DMSO**: Pharmaceutical-grade DMSO should be used to avoid impurities that could harm tissue.

- **Consultation with Healthcare Professionals**: Use of DMSO in wound care should be under the guidance of a qualified healthcare provider to ensure appropriate application and monitoring.

Soft Tissue Injuries

Introduction

Soft tissue injuries refer to damage affecting muscles, ligaments, tendons, and fascia—the non-bony structures that support and move the body's skeletal framework. Common examples include sprains, strains, contusions, and overuse injuries. These injuries are prevalent in both athletic and general populations, often resulting from trauma, repetitive stress, or sudden overexertion. They can lead to pain, swelling, decreased range of motion, and impaired function, impacting an individual's quality of life and ability to perform daily activities.

Dimethyl sulfoxide (DMSO) has been explored as a therapeutic agent for soft tissue injuries due to its anti-inflammatory, analgesic, and membrane-penetrating properties. This section examines the mechanisms by which DMSO may facilitate healing in soft tissue injuries, reviews scientific evidence supporting its use, and discusses practical considerations for clinical application.

Mechanisms of DMSO in Soft Tissue Injury Management

Anti-Inflammatory Effects

- **Modulation of Inflammatory Mediators**: Following soft tissue injury, the body initiates an inflammatory response characterized by the release of pro-inflammatory cytokines such as interleukin-6 (IL-6) and tumor necrosis factor-alpha (TNF-α). DMSO has been shown to inhibit the production and activity of these cytokines, thereby reducing inflammation and associated symptoms like pain and swelling.

- **Inhibition of Leukocyte Migration**: DMSO can impede the migration of neutrophils and macrophages to the injury site. By limiting the accumulation of these inflammatory cells, DMSO reduces the release of enzymes and reactive species that can cause further tissue damage.

Antioxidant Properties

- **Reactive Oxygen Species (ROS) Scavenging**: Injury-induced inflammation often leads to the generation of ROS, which can damage cellular components and exacerbate tissue injury. DMSO acts as a free radical scavenger, neutralizing ROS and protecting tissues from oxidative stress.

Enhancement of Microcirculation

- **Improved Blood Flow**: DMSO may enhance microcirculation within injured tissues by causing vasodilation and reducing blood viscosity. Improved blood flow facilitates the delivery of oxygen and nutrients essential for tissue repair and removes metabolic waste products.

Membrane Penetration and Drug Delivery

- **Transdermal Carrier**: DMSO's ability to penetrate biological membranes allows it to serve as a carrier for other therapeutic agents. When combined with analgesics or anti-inflammatory drugs, DMSO can enhance their delivery to deeper tissues, potentially increasing therapeutic efficacy.

Edema Reduction

- **Decrease in Swelling**: By modulating capillary permeability and reducing inflammation, DMSO can help decrease edema associated with soft tissue injuries, promoting comfort and mobility.

Scientific Evidence and Research Findings

Preclinical Studies

- **Animal Models**: Research using animal models of soft tissue injury, such as induced muscle strains or ligament sprains in rodents, has demonstrated that topical application of DMSO reduces inflammation, minimizes tissue damage, and accelerates functional recovery.

- **Cellular Mechanisms**: In vitro studies have shown that DMSO can modulate signaling pathways involved in inflammation and cell survival, supporting its potential role in enhancing soft tissue healing.

Clinical Studies

- **Sprains and Strains**: Clinical trials involving patients with acute ankle sprains reported that DMSO gel application led to significant reductions in pain and swelling compared to placebo. Patients also experienced improved joint function and faster return to activity.

- **Contusions**: Studies on muscle contusions have indicated that DMSO treatment reduces hematoma size and tenderness, facilitating quicker resolution of bruising.

- **Overuse Injuries**: Athletes with overuse injuries, such as tendinopathies, have reported symptomatic relief with DMSO application, though more rigorous studies are needed to confirm efficacy.

Comparative Studies

- **DMSO vs. Standard Treatments**: Some studies have compared DMSO with standard anti-inflammatory medications like NSAIDs. Results suggest that DMSO may offer comparable benefits with fewer systemic side effects, particularly when used topically.

Limitations

- **Study Quality**: Many existing studies have methodological limitations, including small sample sizes, lack of blinding, and inconsistent dosing protocols.

- **Need for Further Research**: High-quality, randomized controlled trials are necessary to establish definitive evidence for DMSO's effectiveness in soft tissue injuries.

Clinical Applications

Topical Administration

- **Formulations**: DMSO is available in various formulations suitable for topical use, including gels, creams, and solutions. Concentrations ranging from 25% to 70% are commonly used, with higher concentrations potentially offering greater penetration but also increasing the risk of skin irritation.

- **Application Protocol**: The affected area should be cleansed before application to remove any substances that could be carried into the skin by DMSO. A thin layer of DMSO is then applied to the skin overlying the injury, typically two to three times per day.

Combination Therapies

- **Co-administration with Medications**: DMSO can be combined with other topical agents, such as corticosteroids, NSAIDs, or local anesthetics, to enhance their absorption and therapeutic effect.

- **Adjunct to Physical Therapy**: Incorporating DMSO treatment into a comprehensive rehabilitation program may improve outcomes by reducing pain and inflammation, allowing for more effective physical therapy sessions.

Safety and Side Effects

Local Reactions

- **Skin Irritation**: Possible adverse effects include redness, itching, and a burning sensation at the application site. These are generally mild and transient but warrant caution, especially with higher DMSO concentrations.

- **Allergic Reactions**: Although rare, hypersensitivity reactions can occur. A patch test on a small skin area is recommended before widespread application to assess individual tolerance.

Systemic Effects

- **Odor**: A characteristic garlic-like odor on the breath and skin is common due to DMSO's metabolism to dimethyl sulfide. While harmless, this may be unpleasant for some individuals.

- **Systemic Absorption**: DMSO's ability to enhance the absorption of other substances underscores the importance of ensuring that the skin is free from contaminants before application.

Precautions

- **Contraindications**: DMSO should be used cautiously in individuals with known allergies to the compound, during pregnancy or breastfeeding, and in those with severe liver or kidney impairment.

- **Drug Interactions**: Enhanced absorption of concomitant medications may alter their pharmacokinetics and pharmacodynamics, necessitating medical supervision.

Practical Considerations

Patient Assessment

- **Medical Evaluation**: Before initiating DMSO treatment, a thorough medical history and physical examination should be conducted to rule out fractures or more severe injuries requiring different interventions.

- **Individualized Treatment**: Dosage and duration of DMSO therapy should be tailored to the specific injury and patient response.

Application Guidelines

- **Hygiene**: Both the applicator's hands and the application site must be clean to prevent the introduction of pathogens or harmful substances.

- **Protective Measures**: Using gloves during application can prevent self-exposure and minimize the transfer of odor.

- **Follow-Up**: Regular monitoring of the injury's healing progress and any potential side effects is important to adjust treatment as needed.

Patient Education

- **Instructions**: Clear guidance on how to apply DMSO correctly, potential side effects, and signs of adverse reactions ensures safe use.

- **Expectations**: Setting realistic expectations regarding the extent and timeline of symptom improvement can enhance patient satisfaction and adherence to the treatment plan.

Skin Conditions

Introduction

Skin conditions encompass a wide array of disorders affecting the integumentary system, including inflammatory diseases, infections, autoimmune disorders, and neoplastic processes. Common skin conditions such as psoriasis, eczema (atopic dermatitis), acne, rosacea, and scleroderma can significantly impact an individual's quality of life due to symptoms like itching, pain, and cosmetic concerns. Dimethyl sulfoxide (DMSO) has been investigated for its potential therapeutic effects in various skin conditions, attributed to its anti-inflammatory, antimicrobial, antioxidant, and penetration-enhancing properties. This section examines the mechanisms by which DMSO may benefit skin disorders, reviews scientific evidence, and discusses practical considerations for its clinical application.

Mechanisms of DMSO in Skin Conditions

Anti-Inflammatory Effects

- **Cytokine Modulation**: DMSO has been shown to inhibit the production of pro-inflammatory cytokines such as interleukin-1 beta (IL-1β), interleukin-6 (IL-6), and tumor necrosis factor-alpha (TNF-α). By reducing these mediators, DMSO may alleviate inflammatory processes underlying conditions like psoriasis and eczema.

- **Inhibition of Nuclear Factor Kappa B (NF-κB)**: DMSO can suppress the activation of NF-κB, a transcription factor that regulates genes involved in inflammation and immune responses, potentially reducing the severity of inflammatory skin diseases.

Antimicrobial Properties

- **Broad-Spectrum Antimicrobial Activity**: DMSO exhibits antimicrobial effects against various bacteria and fungi. This property may help manage skin infections or secondary infections associated with conditions like acne or eczema.

Antioxidant Activity

- **Reactive Oxygen Species (ROS) Scavenging**: By neutralizing ROS, DMSO may protect skin cells from oxidative stress, which is implicated in the pathogenesis of conditions such as psoriasis and scleroderma.

Penetration Enhancement

- **Transdermal Drug Delivery**: DMSO's ability to penetrate the stratum corneum enhances the delivery of co-administered therapeutic agents, including corticosteroids, antibiotics, and other topical medications used in dermatology.

Modulation of Immune Responses

- **Immunomodulatory Effects**: DMSO may influence immune cell function, potentially benefiting autoimmune skin conditions by modulating aberrant immune responses.

Scientific Evidence and Research Findings

Psoriasis

- **Clinical Studies**: Some studies have explored the use of DMSO as a vehicle for topical medications in psoriasis treatment. DMSO combined with corticosteroids has shown enhanced efficacy compared to corticosteroids alone, possibly due to improved skin penetration.

- **Monotherapy Trials**: Limited trials using DMSO alone have reported reductions in plaque thickness and scaling. However, results are variable, and further research is needed to confirm efficacy.

Eczema (Atopic Dermatitis)

- **Anti-Inflammatory Effects**: Preclinical studies suggest that DMSO's anti-inflammatory properties may alleviate symptoms of eczema. Clinical data are sparse, and more studies are required to establish therapeutic benefits.

Acne Vulgaris

- **Antimicrobial Action**: DMSO's antibacterial properties against *Propionibacterium acnes* (now *Cutibacterium acnes*), the bacteria associated with acne, have been investigated. When used as a solvent for topical antibiotics, DMSO may enhance drug penetration and efficacy.

- **Sebum Regulation**: There is limited evidence on DMSO's effect on sebum production. Its role in acne management primarily revolves around improving the delivery of anti-acne agents.

Scleroderma

- **Skin Softening**: DMSO has been studied for its potential to soften skin in patients with localized scleroderma (morphea) due to its collagen-modulating effects.

- **Clinical Trials**: Early studies reported improvements in skin pliability and reduction of induration with topical DMSO application. However, these findings are preliminary, and larger controlled studies are necessary.

Herpes Simplex Infections

- **Antiviral Delivery**: DMSO has been used as a vehicle to enhance the penetration of antiviral medications like acyclovir for treating herpes simplex lesions.

- **Symptom Relief**: Some patients reported faster lesion resolution and reduced pain when DMSO was included in topical formulations, though evidence is anecdotal.

Limitations of Current Research

- **Study Quality**: Many studies are limited by small sample sizes, lack of controls, and inconsistent methodologies.

- **Need for Rigorous Trials**: High-quality randomized controlled trials are essential to establish the safety and efficacy of DMSO in various skin conditions conclusively.

Clinical Applications

Topical Administration

- **Formulations**: DMSO is applied topically in concentrations typically ranging from 30% to 70%, depending on the condition and patient tolerance.

- **Combination Therapies**: DMSO is often used as a solvent or vehicle to enhance the delivery of other topical medications, such as corticosteroids, antifungals, or retinoids.

Application Protocols

- **Frequency**: Application frequency varies but generally ranges from once to multiple times daily, as directed by a healthcare professional.

- **Skin Preparation**: The skin should be clean and dry before application to prevent unintended absorption of contaminants.

Safety and Side Effects

Local Adverse Effects

- **Skin Irritation**: Common side effects include redness, itching, burning sensation, and dryness at the application site. These are usually mild and transient.

- **Contact Dermatitis**: Allergic reactions can occur, though they are relatively rare. A patch test may be advisable before widespread use.

- **Photosensitivity**: DMSO may increase skin sensitivity to sunlight; patients should be advised to use sun protection.

Systemic Effects

- **Odor**: DMSO metabolism can produce a garlic-like odor on the breath and skin, which may be bothersome but is harmless.

- **Systemic Absorption**: While systemic absorption from topical application is generally low, DMSO can enhance the absorption of other substances, necessitating caution.

Precautions

- **Contraindications**: DMSO should be used cautiously in individuals with known hypersensitivity, during pregnancy or breastfeeding, and in those with significant liver or kidney impairment.

- **Drug Interactions**: Enhanced absorption of concomitant medications may alter their effects; medical supervision is recommended.

Chronic Conditions

Introduction

Chronic conditions are long-lasting diseases or health issues that persist for extended periods, often impacting an individual's quality of life and requiring ongoing medical attention. These conditions can be complex, involving multifaceted pathophysiological processes that make management challenging. Dimethyl sulfoxide (DMSO) has been explored for its potential therapeutic applications in various chronic diseases due to its anti-inflammatory, immunomodulatory, and antioxidant properties. This section examines the scientific basis for using DMSO in chronic conditions, reviews relevant clinical evidence, and discusses practical considerations for its use under medical supervision.

Mechanisms of Action in Chronic Conditions

Anti-Inflammatory Effects

- **Cytokine Suppression**: DMSO inhibits the production of pro-inflammatory cytokines such as interleukin-1 beta (IL-1β) and tumor necrosis factor-alpha (TNF-α), which play significant roles in chronic inflammatory processes.

- **Inhibition of NF-κB Pathway**: By suppressing the activation of nuclear factor kappa B (NF-κB), DMSO reduces the transcription of genes involved in chronic inflammation.

Immunomodulatory Properties

- **Regulation of Immune Cells**: DMSO modulates the function of various immune cells, including T cells and macrophages, potentially restoring immune balance in autoimmune conditions.

- **Antibody Production**: It may influence the production of autoantibodies, which are implicated in several chronic autoimmune diseases.

Antioxidant Activities

- **Reactive Oxygen Species Scavenging**: DMSO neutralizes reactive oxygen species (ROS), reducing oxidative stress that contributes to the progression of chronic diseases.

- **Protection Against Lipid Peroxidation**: By preventing lipid peroxidation in cell membranes, DMSO preserves cellular integrity and function.

Enhancement of Cellular Metabolism

- **Mitochondrial Support**: DMSO may improve mitochondrial function, enhancing cellular energy production and reducing metabolic dysfunction associated with chronic conditions.

Potential Therapeutic Applications

Interstitial Cystitis

- **FDA-Approved Use**: DMSO is approved by the U.S. Food and Drug Administration (FDA) for intravesical instillation in the treatment of interstitial cystitis, a chronic inflammatory condition of the bladder.

- **Mechanism of Action**: DMSO is believed to reduce bladder inflammation by decreasing nerve hyperactivity, modulating mast cell activity, and enhancing the integrity of the bladder's glycosaminoglycan layer.

- **Clinical Evidence**: Studies have shown that DMSO instillation can alleviate pain, reduce urinary frequency, and improve bladder capacity in patients with interstitial cystitis.

Scleroderma

- **Skin Softening Effects**: DMSO has been investigated for its potential to improve skin elasticity in scleroderma, a chronic autoimmune disease characterized by skin thickening due to excessive collagen deposition.

- **Collagen Modulation**: It may inhibit fibroblast proliferation and collagen synthesis, reducing skin fibrosis.

- **Clinical Studies**: Some patients treated with topical DMSO reported increased skin softness and decreased joint stiffness, although results are variable and require further validation.

Fibromyalgia

- **Pain Reduction**: Fibromyalgia is a chronic condition marked by widespread musculoskeletal pain. DMSO's analgesic and anti-inflammatory properties might offer symptom relief.

- **Muscle Relaxation**: By modulating nerve conduction and reducing muscle inflammation, DMSO may alleviate muscle tenderness associated with fibromyalgia.

82

- **Evidence**: Limited clinical data are available, and more rigorous studies are needed to establish efficacy.

Autoimmune Diseases

- **Rheumatoid Arthritis**: Beyond its use in pain management, DMSO's immunomodulatory effects could potentially slow disease progression by modulating immune responses.

- **Systemic Lupus Erythematosus (SLE)**: DMSO may reduce autoantibody production and inflammatory cytokine levels, although clinical evidence is sparse.

- **Multiple Sclerosis**: Preliminary research suggests DMSO might have neuroprotective effects, but conclusive clinical trials are lacking.

Neurodegenerative Diseases

- **Antioxidant Protection**: DMSO's ability to scavenge free radicals may protect neuronal cells from oxidative damage implicated in diseases like Alzheimer's and Parkinson's.

- **Anti-Aggregation Effects**: It may inhibit the aggregation of misfolded proteins, a hallmark of certain neurodegenerative disorders.

- **Research Status**: Most studies are preclinical, and significant research is required to determine therapeutic potential in humans.

Clinical Evidence and Research Findings

Interstitial Cystitis Studies

- **Efficacy Demonstrated**: Multiple clinical trials have supported the use of intravesical DMSO in improving symptoms of interstitial cystitis.

- **Long-Term Benefits**: Some patients experience sustained relief with periodic treatments.

Scleroderma Research

- **Mixed Results**: Clinical trials have produced inconsistent findings regarding DMSO's effectiveness in scleroderma, highlighting the need for further investigation.

Other Chronic Conditions

- **Limited Data**: For fibromyalgia, autoimmune diseases, and neurodegenerative disorders, clinical evidence is limited or preliminary.

- **Need for Rigorous Trials**: High-quality randomized controlled trials are essential to establish the safety and efficacy of DMSO in these conditions.

Safety and Side Effects

General Safety Profile

- **Adverse Effects**: Common side effects include skin irritation, itching, and a garlic-like odor due to dimethyl sulfide formation.

- **Systemic Effects**: Oral or intravenous use may cause gastrointestinal disturbances, headache, dizziness, or allergic reactions.

Long-Term Use Considerations

- **Organ Toxicity**: Prolonged use at high doses may pose risks to liver and kidney function; monitoring is recommended.

- **Reproductive Effects**: Animal studies suggest potential teratogenic effects; DMSO should be used cautiously in pregnant or breastfeeding women.

Monitoring Requirements

- **Regular Assessments**: Patients undergoing long-term DMSO therapy should have periodic evaluations of organ function and overall health status.

- **Dose Adjustments**: Dosing may need to be modified based on therapeutic response and the occurrence of side effects.

Practical Considerations

Guidelines for Use Under Medical Supervision

- **Professional Oversight**: DMSO should be administered under the guidance of a qualified healthcare provider, especially for chronic conditions.

- **Individualized Treatment Plans**: Therapy should be tailored to the patient's specific condition, severity, and response to treatment.

Dosing Considerations

- **Route of Administration**: Depends on the condition—intravesical for interstitial cystitis, topical for scleroderma, and investigational routes for other conditions.

- **Dosage Regimens**: Should follow established protocols where available; otherwise, dosing should be based on clinical judgment and patient tolerance.

Patient Selection and Contraindications

- **Candidate Evaluation**: Assess for contraindications such as hypersensitivity to DMSO, significant organ dysfunction, or concurrent medications that may interact.

- **Informed Consent**: Patients should be informed about potential benefits, risks, and the experimental nature of some treatments.

Interstitial Cystitis

Introduction

Interstitial cystitis (IC), also known as bladder pain syndrome (BPS), is a chronic condition characterized by pelvic pain, urinary urgency, frequency, and discomfort associated with bladder filling. The etiology of IC remains unclear, but it is believed to involve a combination of factors such as epithelial dysfunction, mast cell activation, neurogenic inflammation, and autoimmune responses. The condition predominantly affects women and can significantly impair quality of life due to persistent symptoms and associated psychological distress.

Dimethyl sulfoxide (DMSO) is the only intravesical therapy approved by the U.S. Food and Drug Administration (FDA) specifically for the treatment of interstitial cystitis. This section explores the role of DMSO in managing IC, focusing on its mechanisms of action, clinical efficacy, administration protocols, safety considerations, and future research directions.

Pathophysiology of Interstitial Cystitis

Interstitial cystitis is a multifactorial disorder involving complex interactions between the bladder epithelium, immune system, and nervous system:

- **Epithelial Dysfunction**: Damage to the glycosaminoglycan (GAG) layer of the bladder mucosa increases permeability, allowing urinary solutes to penetrate and irritate underlying tissues.

- **Mast Cell Activation**: Increased numbers of activated mast cells release histamine and other inflammatory mediators, contributing to pain and inflammation.

- **Neurogenic Inflammation**: Sensory nerve fibers release neuropeptides like substance P, leading to heightened pain perception and further inflammation.

- **Autoimmune Components**: Some patients exhibit autoimmune responses, with antibodies targeting bladder antigens.

Mechanisms of DMSO in Interstitial Cystitis Management

DMSO exerts multiple therapeutic effects that address key aspects of IC pathophysiology:

Anti-Inflammatory Actions

- **Mast Cell Inhibition**: DMSO stabilizes mast cells, reducing the release of histamine and other pro-inflammatory mediators.

- **Cytokine Modulation**: It decreases the production of pro-inflammatory cytokines, mitigating inflammation within the bladder wall.

Analgesic Effects

- **Nerve Conduction Modulation**: DMSO may interrupt C-fiber nerve transmission, diminishing pain signals associated with bladder filling and urination.

- **Neurotransmitter Regulation**: It influences the levels of neurotransmitters involved in pain perception, potentially reducing hypersensitivity.

Muscle Relaxation

- **Smooth Muscle Effects**: DMSO can induce relaxation of bladder smooth muscle, alleviating symptoms of urinary urgency and frequency.

Enhancement of Bladder Mucosal Integrity

- **GAG Layer Restoration**: By penetrating the bladder wall, DMSO may promote healing of the urothelium and restoration of the protective GAG layer.

Antimicrobial Properties

- **Infection Prevention**: Although not primarily an antimicrobial agent, DMSO's ability to inhibit bacterial growth may reduce secondary infections that can exacerbate IC symptoms.

Clinical Evidence and Research Findings

Efficacy Studies

- **Randomized Controlled Trials**: Clinical trials have demonstrated that intravesical DMSO therapy leads to significant improvement in pain relief, urinary frequency, and bladder capacity compared to placebo.

- **Long-Term Benefits**: Some patients experience sustained symptom relief for several months after a course of DMSO treatments.

- **Response Rates**: Approximately 50–70% of patients report symptom improvement following DMSO therapy.

Comparative Studies

- **Versus Other Treatments**: Studies comparing DMSO with other intravesical agents like hyaluronic acid or heparin show that DMSO is similarly effective or superior in symptom reduction.

- **Combination Therapies**: Combining DMSO with other agents such as steroids or anesthetics may enhance therapeutic outcomes, though more research is needed.

Mechanistic Studies

- **Biopsy Analysis**: Bladder biopsies from patients treated with DMSO show reduced inflammation and mast cell counts.

- **Urodynamic Studies**: Improvements in bladder compliance and capacity have been observed after DMSO treatment.

Administration Protocols

Intravesical Instillation Procedure

- **Preparation**: The bladder is emptied before instillation. A catheter is inserted aseptically into the bladder.

- **DMSO Solution**: A 50% aqueous solution of pharmaceutical-grade DMSO is typically used.

- **Instillation Volume**: Approximately 50 mL of the DMSO solution is instilled into the bladder.

- **Dwell Time**: The solution is retained in the bladder for about 15–20 minutes, although some protocols allow up to one hour if tolerated.

- **Frequency**: Treatments are usually administered once weekly for 6–8 weeks. Maintenance therapy may be individualized based on patient response.

- **Post-Procedure Care**: Patients are advised to monitor for side effects and report any significant discomfort.

Combination with Other Agents

- **Anesthetics**: Lidocaine may be added to reduce discomfort during instillation.

- **Anti-Inflammatory Drugs**: Steroids or heparin can be combined with DMSO to enhance anti-inflammatory effects.

Safety and Side Effects

Common Adverse Effects

- **Bladder Irritation**: Some patients experience transient bladder discomfort, burning sensations, or spasms during or after instillation.

- **Odor**: A garlic-like taste or odor on the breath and skin may occur for up to 72 hours due to DMSO metabolism to dimethyl sulfide.

- **Urinary Frequency**: Temporary increases in urinary urgency or frequency may be noted following treatment.

Less Common Adverse Effects

- **Allergic Reactions**: Rare cases of hypersensitivity to DMSO have been reported, necessitating discontinuation.

- **Gastrointestinal Symptoms**: Nausea or abdominal cramps may occur but are typically mild.

Safety Precautions

- **Pregnancy and Lactation**: DMSO is classified as a pregnancy category C drug. Its use should be considered only if the potential benefits justify the potential risks.

- **Concurrent Medications**: Patients should inform their healthcare provider of all medications they are taking, as DMSO may enhance the absorption of other drugs.

Monitoring

- **Symptom Evaluation**: Regular assessment of symptom severity and bladder function is essential to gauge treatment efficacy.

- **Adverse Effects**: Patients should be monitored for side effects, and dose adjustments should be made accordingly.

Practical Considerations

Patient Selection

- **Diagnosis Confirmation**: Accurate diagnosis of interstitial cystitis is crucial, often involving cystoscopy and exclusion of other urinary tract disorders.

- **Assessment of Severity**: Evaluating symptom severity helps tailor the treatment regimen to the individual patient.

Informed Consent

- **Explanation of Procedure**: Patients should be thoroughly informed about the instillation process, potential benefits, and possible side effects.

- **Expectations Management**: Setting realistic expectations regarding symptom improvement and treatment duration enhances patient satisfaction.

Multidisciplinary Approach

- **Adjunct Therapies**: Combining DMSO treatment with dietary modifications, physical therapy, and behavioral interventions may improve outcomes.

- **Follow-Up Care**: Regular follow-up appointments are necessary to adjust treatment plans and address any concerns.

Fibromyalgia

Introduction

Fibromyalgia is a chronic disorder characterized by widespread musculoskeletal pain, fatigue, sleep disturbances, cognitive dysfunction, and heightened sensitivity to stimuli. Affecting approximately 2–4% of the global population—predominantly women—fibromyalgia significantly impairs quality of life and functional capacity. The etiology of fibromyalgia is multifactorial, involving abnormalities in pain processing pathways, neurotransmitter imbalances, hormonal dysregulation, and genetic predispositions. Conventional treatments focus on symptom management through pharmacological interventions, physical therapy, and psychological support. Dimethyl sulfoxide (DMSO) has emerged as a potential adjunct therapy due to its analgesic, anti-inflammatory, and neuromodulatory properties. This section explores the scientific rationale for DMSO's use in fibromyalgia, reviews current research findings, and discusses practical considerations for clinical application.

Pathophysiology of Fibromyalgia

Fibromyalgia's complex pathophysiology involves several interconnected mechanisms:

- **Central Sensitization**: Enhanced excitability of neurons in the central nervous system leads to amplified pain signals, resulting in allodynia (pain from non-painful stimuli) and hyperalgesia (increased pain from painful stimuli).

- **Neurotransmitter Imbalance**: Altered levels of serotonin, norepinephrine, dopamine, and substance P affect pain modulation, mood regulation, and stress responses.

- **Hypothalamic-Pituitary-Adrenal (HPA) Axis Dysfunction**: Impaired stress response mechanisms contribute to fatigue, sleep disturbances, and hormonal imbalances.

- **Autonomic Nervous System Dysregulation**: Abnormalities in autonomic function may cause symptoms like irritable bowel syndrome, orthostatic hypotension, and temperature sensitivity.

- **Genetic and Environmental Factors**: Genetic predisposition combined with environmental triggers such as infections or physical/emotional trauma may initiate or exacerbate the condition.

Potential Mechanisms of DMSO in Fibromyalgia Management

Analgesic Effects

- **Modulation of Pain Pathways**: DMSO may influence ion channels and neurotransmitter systems involved in nociception, potentially reducing neuronal hyperexcitability.

- **Peripheral Nerve Impact**: By stabilizing neuronal membranes and decreasing ectopic discharges, DMSO could alleviate peripheral pain signals contributing to central sensitization.

Anti-Inflammatory Actions

- **Cytokine Inhibition**: DMSO suppresses pro-inflammatory cytokines like interleukin-6 (IL-6) and tumor necrosis factor-alpha (TNF-α), which are elevated in some fibromyalgia patients.

- **Oxidative Stress Reduction**: Its antioxidant properties help neutralize reactive oxygen species (ROS), mitigating oxidative damage associated with chronic pain and fatigue.

Neuromodulatory Effects

- **Neurotransmitter Regulation**: DMSO may affect the synthesis and release of neurotransmitters involved in pain perception and mood, such as serotonin and substance P.

- **Glial Cell Interaction**: By modulating glial cell activity, DMSO might reduce neuroinflammation and neuronal sensitization.

Muscle Relaxation and Microcirculation Enhancement

- **Vasodilation**: DMSO-induced vasodilation can improve blood flow to muscles, enhancing oxygen and nutrient delivery and facilitating the removal of metabolic waste.

- **Muscle Fiber Effects**: It may decrease muscle stiffness and spasms by affecting muscle fiber contractility and reducing inflammation.

Clinical Evidence and Research Findings

Clinical Studies

- **Limited Human Trials**: There is a scarcity of robust clinical trials investigating DMSO's efficacy in fibromyalgia. Existing studies often have small sample sizes and lack rigorous design.

- **Symptom Improvement Reports**: Some patients report reductions in pain intensity, improved sleep quality, and enhanced overall well-being with DMSO use, but these findings are largely anecdotal.

Preclinical Research

- **Animal Models**: Studies using animal models of chronic pain demonstrate that DMSO can reduce pain behaviors and inflammatory markers, supporting its potential analgesic effects.

- **Cellular Studies**: In vitro research shows that DMSO can modulate inflammatory pathways and oxidative stress, which are relevant to fibromyalgia pathology.

Combination Therapies

- **Adjunctive Use**: DMSO has been studied in combination with other agents like magnesium sulfate and lidocaine, showing potential synergistic effects in pain reduction.

- **Transdermal Delivery**: Its penetration-enhancing properties facilitate the transdermal administration of other medications, potentially improving therapeutic outcomes.

Limitations of Current Research

- **Methodological Issues**: Many studies lack control groups, have short durations, and use subjective outcome measures.

- **Need for Comprehensive Trials**: Rigorous randomized controlled trials are essential to establish definitive efficacy and safety profiles.

Administration Methods

Topical Application

- **Formulations**: DMSO is available in gels, creams, and liquid solutions, typically in concentrations ranging from 25% to 70%.

- **Application Sites**: Applied directly to areas of musculoskeletal pain, such as the neck, shoulders, back, and extremities.

- **Dosage and Frequency**: Standard practice involves applying a thin layer two to three times daily, with adjustments based on patient response and tolerance.

Oral Administration

- **Systemic Effects**: Oral DMSO is less commonly used due to potential gastrointestinal side effects and limited evidence of efficacy in fibromyalgia.

- **Dosing Considerations**: If considered, it should be under strict medical supervision, with careful dosing to minimize adverse effects.

Combination with Other Therapies

- **Pharmacological Agents**: DMSO may enhance the efficacy of co-administered topical medications like NSAIDs or analgesics.

- **Non-Pharmacological Interventions**: Incorporating DMSO into a multimodal treatment plan that includes physical therapy, cognitive-behavioral therapy, and lifestyle modifications may offer additional benefits.

Safety and Side Effects

Local Adverse Effects

- **Skin Irritation**: Common side effects include redness, dryness, itching, and a burning sensation at the application site.

- **Allergic Reactions**: Although rare, hypersensitivity reactions can occur; a patch test is recommended before widespread use.

Systemic Adverse Effects

- **Odor**: DMSO metabolism produces dimethyl sulfide, causing a transient garlic-like odor on the breath and skin.

- **Gastrointestinal Symptoms**: Oral administration may lead to nausea, vomiting, diarrhea, and abdominal cramps.

Precautions and Contraindications

- **Pregnancy and Lactation**: The safety of DMSO during pregnancy and breastfeeding is not established; it should be avoided unless deemed necessary by a healthcare provider.

- **Renal and Hepatic Impairment**: Patients with kidney or liver dysfunction should use DMSO cautiously, as these organs are involved in its excretion and metabolism.

- **Drug Interactions**: DMSO may enhance the absorption of other medications, potentially leading to increased effects or toxicity.

Practical Considerations

Patient Selection

- **Comprehensive Assessment**: A thorough evaluation to confirm the fibromyalgia diagnosis and assess symptom severity is essential.

- **Individualized Approach**: Treatment should be tailored to the patient's specific symptoms, preferences, and comorbidities.

Application Guidelines

- **Skin Preparation**: Ensure the application area is clean and free from other substances that could be absorbed.

- **Instruction and Education**: Provide detailed guidance on proper application techniques, dosage, and potential side effects.

- **Monitoring**: Regular follow-up to evaluate efficacy, adherence, and any adverse reactions.

Multidisciplinary Collaboration

- **Integrated Care**: Collaboration among rheumatologists, pain specialists, physical therapists, and mental health professionals can optimize treatment outcomes.

- **Patient Empowerment**: Encouraging patient involvement in decision-making and self-management strategies enhances engagement and satisfaction.

Introduction

Autoimmune disorders occur when the immune system mistakenly attacks the body's own tissues, leading to chronic inflammation and tissue damage. These conditions encompass a wide range of diseases, including rheumatoid arthritis, systemic lupus erythematosus, multiple sclerosis, and psoriasis. Autoimmune diseases can affect various organs and systems, resulting in significant morbidity and a decreased quality of life. The complexity of their pathogenesis makes treatment challenging, often requiring long-term immunosuppressive therapy with potential side effects. Dimethyl sulfoxide (DMSO) has been investigated as a potential therapeutic agent in autoimmune disorders due to its anti-inflammatory, immunomodulatory, and antioxidant properties. This section explores the scientific rationale for using DMSO in autoimmune diseases, reviews relevant research findings, and discusses practical considerations for its clinical application.

Pathophysiology of Autoimmune Disorders

Autoimmune diseases are characterized by a loss of immunological tolerance, where the immune system fails to recognize self-antigens and initiates an attack against the body's own cells and tissues. Key features include:

- **Aberrant Immune Responses**: Activation of autoreactive T and B lymphocytes leads to the production of autoantibodies and cytotoxic T cells that target specific tissues.

- **Cytokine Dysregulation**: An imbalance of pro-inflammatory and anti-inflammatory cytokines contributes to chronic inflammation and tissue destruction.

- **Genetic and Environmental Factors**: Genetic predisposition combined with environmental triggers such as infections or toxins can initiate or exacerbate autoimmune processes.

- **Molecular Mimicry**: Pathogens may possess antigens similar to self-antigens, leading to cross-reactivity and autoimmunity.

Potential Mechanisms of DMSO in Autoimmune Disease Management

Immunomodulatory Effects

- **Regulation of Lymphocyte Function**: DMSO may modulate the activity of T helper cells and cytotoxic T cells, reducing the proliferation of autoreactive lymphocytes.

- **Cytokine Modulation**: By inhibiting the production of pro-inflammatory cytokines like interleukin-1 beta (IL-1β), interleukin-6 (IL-6), and tumor necrosis factor-alpha (TNF-α), DMSO can shift the immune response towards a less inflammatory profile.

- **Suppression of Autoantibody Production**: DMSO might decrease B cell activity and autoantibody synthesis, potentially reducing immune complex formation and tissue damage.

Anti-Inflammatory Actions

- **Inhibition of Inflammatory Pathways**: DMSO can suppress the activation of nuclear factor kappa B (NF-κB), a key transcription factor involved in the expression of inflammatory genes.

- **Reduction of Oxidative Stress**: Its antioxidant properties help scavenge reactive oxygen species (ROS), mitigating oxidative damage associated with chronic inflammation.

Tissue Protection and Repair

- **Membrane Stabilization**: DMSO may protect cells by stabilizing cell membranes and preserving cellular integrity.

- **Promotion of Healing Processes**: By enhancing microcirculation and reducing fibrosis, DMSO could support tissue repair in affected organs.

Clinical Evidence and Research Findings

Rheumatoid Arthritis (RA)

- **Preclinical Studies**: Animal models of RA have demonstrated that DMSO administration reduces joint inflammation, pannus formation, and cartilage erosion. DMSO's effects were attributed to decreased cytokine production and inhibition of inflammatory cell infiltration.

- **Clinical Observations**: Some early clinical trials reported that topical DMSO application led to modest improvements in pain, swelling, and joint stiffness in RA patients. However, results were inconsistent, and side effects such as skin irritation limited its use.

- **Limitations**: The lack of large-scale, placebo-controlled studies makes it difficult to draw definitive conclusions about DMSO's efficacy in RA.

Systemic Lupus Erythematosus (SLE)

- **Mechanistic Insights**: In vitro studies suggest that DMSO can inhibit lymphocyte proliferation and reduce the production of autoantibodies involved in SLE pathogenesis.

- **Clinical Data**: Clinical evidence is sparse, with few case reports indicating potential benefits in reducing disease activity. More rigorous studies are needed to evaluate therapeutic potential.

Multiple Sclerosis (MS)

- **Neuroprotective Potential**: DMSO's antioxidant and anti-inflammatory properties may offer neuroprotection by reducing demyelination and axonal damage.

- **Animal Studies**: Experimental autoimmune encephalomyelitis (EAE) models have shown that DMSO treatment decreases neurological deficits and inflammation in the central nervous system.

- **Human Studies**: Clinical trials are limited, and existing studies do not provide sufficient evidence to support DMSO use in MS patients.

Psoriasis

- **Topical Application**: DMSO has been used as a solvent to enhance the penetration of therapeutic agents like corticosteroids and methotrexate in psoriasis treatment.

- **Direct Effects**: Some studies suggest that DMSO alone may reduce plaque thickness and scaling due to its anti-inflammatory actions, but evidence is limited and inconclusive.

Limitations Across Studies

- **Heterogeneity**: Variability in study designs, patient populations, DMSO concentrations, and administration routes complicates data interpretation.

- **Small Sample Sizes**: Many studies involve a limited number of participants, reducing statistical power.

- **Need for Standardization**: Consistent methodologies are necessary to compare results and establish definitive conclusions.

Administration Methods

Topical Application

- **Formulations**: DMSO is applied as creams, gels, or ointments, typically in concentrations of 50–70%, depending on the condition and patient tolerance.

- **Application Sites**: For conditions like RA and psoriasis, DMSO is applied directly to affected joints or skin lesions.

- **Frequency**: The frequency of application varies but is commonly two to three times daily.

Oral Administration

- **Systemic Effects**: Oral DMSO has been explored for systemic autoimmune diseases but is limited by potential gastrointestinal side effects and lack of robust clinical evidence.

- **Dosage**: Oral dosing requires careful consideration and should only be undertaken under medical supervision.

Intravenous Administration

- **Experimental Use**: Intravenous DMSO has been used in some research settings but is not standard practice due to concerns about safety and insufficient data on efficacy.

Combination Therapies

- **Enhanced Drug Delivery**: DMSO's penetration-enhancing properties can improve the efficacy of topical medications used in autoimmune conditions.

- **Adjunctive Therapy**: It may be combined with other immunosuppressive agents to potentially enhance therapeutic outcomes.

Safety and Side Effects

Local Adverse Effects

- **Skin Irritation**: Redness, itching, dryness, and a burning sensation may occur at the application site.

- **Dermatitis**: Prolonged use or high concentrations can lead to contact dermatitis in sensitive individuals.

- **Allergic Reactions**: Hypersensitivity reactions are rare but require immediate discontinuation of DMSO.

Systemic Adverse Effects

- **Odor**: A garlic-like odor on the breath and skin is common due to DMSO metabolism to dimethyl sulfide.

- **Gastrointestinal Symptoms**: Oral administration may cause nausea, vomiting, diarrhea, and abdominal discomfort.

- **Neurological Effects**: High doses have been associated with headache, dizziness, and sedation.

Precautions

- **Pregnancy and Lactation**: DMSO is not recommended due to insufficient safety data and potential teratogenic effects observed in animal studies.

- **Organ Dysfunction**: Use with caution in patients with liver or kidney impairment.

- **Drug Interactions**: DMSO may enhance the absorption of other medications, potentially leading to increased effects or toxicity.

Practical Considerations

Patient Assessment

- **Medical Evaluation**: A thorough assessment to confirm the autoimmune diagnosis and evaluate disease severity is essential.

- **Contraindications**: Identify any contraindications or potential interactions with current medications.

Treatment Planning

- **Individualized Approach**: Tailor the treatment regimen to the patient's specific condition, symptoms, and response to therapy.

- **Monitoring**: Regular follow-up to assess efficacy, adjust dosing, and monitor for adverse effects.

Patient Education

- **Informed Consent**: Discuss the experimental nature of DMSO use in autoimmune disorders, including potential benefits and risks.

- **Application Instructions**: Provide clear guidance on proper application techniques and precautions to minimize side effects.

DMSO in Cancer Care

Introduction

Cancer remains a leading cause of mortality worldwide, prompting continuous exploration of novel therapeutic agents and strategies. Dimethyl sulfoxide (DMSO) has attracted scientific interest in oncology due to its unique chemical properties and potential biological activities that may influence cancer cell behavior. This section examines current research on the role of DMSO in cancer care, discussing its mechanisms of action, potential therapeutic applications, and emphasizing the critical need for medical supervision when considering its use.

Potential Mechanisms of Action in Cancer

Modulation of Cell Differentiation

- **Induction of Differentiation**: DMSO has been shown to induce differentiation in certain malignant cells, particularly in leukemic cell lines. By promoting maturation, DMSO may reduce the proliferation rate of these cells and alter their phenotype to resemble normal cells more closely.

Antiproliferative Effects

- **Cell Cycle Arrest**: Research indicates that DMSO can cause cell cycle arrest at specific phases, such as the G1/G0 phase, inhibiting cancer cell division and growth.

- **Apoptosis Induction**: DMSO may trigger programmed cell death in cancer cells through the activation of apoptotic pathways, potentially reducing tumor mass.

Enhancement of Chemotherapy Efficacy

- **Synergistic Effects with Anticancer Drugs**: Studies suggest that DMSO can enhance the effectiveness of certain chemotherapeutic agents by increasing their penetration into cancer cells or by modulating cellular responses to these drugs.

- **Overcoming Drug Resistance**: DMSO may sensitize resistant cancer cells to chemotherapy by affecting membrane permeability and drug efflux mechanisms.

Antioxidant and Free Radical Scavenging

- **Reduction of Oxidative Stress**: While oxidative stress can induce cancer cell death, it may also promote tumor progression and resistance. DMSO's antioxidant properties might protect normal cells during chemotherapy while selectively affecting cancer cells.

Current Research Findings

Preclinical Studies

- **In Vitro Experiments**: Laboratory studies have demonstrated that DMSO can inhibit the growth of various cancer cell types, including leukemia, lymphoma, breast, prostate, and colon cancer cells.

    - *Example*: In human leukemia cell lines, DMSO induced differentiation and decreased proliferation rates.

- **Animal Models**: In vivo studies using mouse models have reported that DMSO administration can reduce tumor growth and enhance the antitumor effects of chemotherapeutic agents like cisplatin and doxorubicin.

Clinical Studies

- **Limited Human Trials**: Clinical research on DMSO in cancer patients is scarce and primarily involves case reports or small pilot studies.

    - *Example*: A pilot study investigating DMSO as a solvent for chemotherapy drugs reported improved drug tolerance but did not provide conclusive evidence of enhanced efficacy.

- **Topical Applications**: In cases of cutaneous metastases, DMSO has been used experimentally as a vehicle for topical chemotherapy, but data are limited and inconclusive.

Challenges and Limitations

- **Inconsistent Results**: Variability in study design, cancer types, DMSO concentrations, and administration routes makes it difficult to draw definitive conclusions.

- **Lack of Large-Scale Clinical Trials**: The absence of robust clinical data limits the ability to assess the true therapeutic potential and safety profile of DMSO in cancer care.

Potential Therapeutic Applications Under Investigation
Leukemia and Lymphoma

- **Differentiation Therapy**: DMSO's capacity to induce differentiation in hematopoietic malignancies presents a potential therapeutic avenue, particularly in acute promyelocytic leukemia (APL).

- **Combination Treatments**: Research is exploring DMSO in combination with agents like all-trans retinoic acid (ATRA) to enhance differentiation and apoptosis in leukemic cells.

Solid Tumors

- **Enhancement of Drug Delivery**: DMSO may improve the delivery and efficacy of chemotherapeutic agents in solid tumors by increasing cell membrane permeability.

- **Sensitization to Radiotherapy**: Preliminary studies suggest that DMSO might sensitize tumor cells to radiation, potentially improving radiotherapy outcomes.

Multidrug Resistance

- **Modulation of Drug Transporters**: DMSO may inhibit the function of P-glycoprotein and other efflux pumps that contribute to chemotherapy resistance, enhancing drug accumulation in cancer cells.

Safety Considerations

Potential Side Effects

- **Cytotoxicity to Normal Cells**: High concentrations of DMSO can be toxic to healthy cells, leading to adverse effects on normal tissues.

- **Organ Toxicity**: Prolonged or excessive use may result in hepatotoxicity, nephrotoxicity, or neurotoxicity.

- **Gastrointestinal Symptoms**: Oral or systemic administration can cause nausea, vomiting, and diarrhea.

- **Allergic Reactions**: Rare hypersensitivity reactions may occur, necessitating immediate medical attention.

Interactions with Conventional Therapies

- **Altered Drug Metabolism**: DMSO may affect the metabolism of chemotherapeutic agents, potentially leading to increased toxicity or reduced efficacy.

- **Unpredictable Pharmacodynamics**: The impact of DMSO on drug distribution and action requires careful consideration to avoid adverse interactions.

Necessity for Medical Supervision

- **Professional Oversight**: Any use of DMSO in cancer treatment should be conducted under the guidance of an oncologist familiar with its properties and potential risks.

- **Individualized Risk Assessment**: Patients require thorough evaluation to determine if the potential benefits outweigh the risks in their specific case.

- **Monitoring**: Regular monitoring for side effects and treatment efficacy is essential to ensure patient safety.

Radiation Protection
Introduction

Exposure to ionizing radiation poses significant risks to biological systems, leading to cellular damage, genetic mutations, and increased risk of cancer. Radiation-induced damage is primarily mediated through the generation of reactive oxygen species (ROS) and free radicals, which can cause oxidative stress and disrupt cellular components such as DNA, proteins, and lipids. The search for effective radioprotective agents has been an area of active research, aiming to mitigate the harmful effects of radiation in medical settings, occupational exposure, and potential nuclear incidents.

Dimethyl sulfoxide (DMSO) has been investigated for its potential radioprotective properties due to its antioxidant capacity and ability to scavenge free radicals. This section explores the mechanisms by which DMSO may confer radiation protection, reviews scientific evidence from preclinical studies, discusses potential applications, and addresses safety considerations.

Mechanisms of Radioprotection by DMSO

Free Radical Scavenging

- **Antioxidant Activity**: DMSO is known for its ability to scavenge free radicals, particularly hydroxyl radicals (•OH), which are highly reactive species generated during ionizing radiation exposure.
- **Reduction of Oxidative Stress**: By neutralizing ROS, DMSO can reduce oxidative damage to cellular components, potentially preserving cell viability and function after radiation exposure.

Protection of DNA Integrity

- **Prevention of DNA Strand Breaks**: DMSO may protect DNA by inhibiting the formation of radiation-induced single and double-strand breaks, thereby reducing mutagenesis and carcinogenesis risk.
- **Stabilization of DNA Structure**: It may interact with DNA molecules to stabilize their structure against the disruptive effects of radiation.

Membrane Stabilization

- **Protection of Cellular Membranes**: DMSO can reduce lipid peroxidation in cell membranes, maintaining membrane integrity and preventing leakage of cellular contents.
- **Preservation of Organelle Function**: By protecting mitochondrial membranes, DMSO may help sustain energy production and apoptotic regulation post-radiation.

Modulation of Cell Signaling Pathways

- **Inhibition of Apoptosis**: DMSO may modulate signaling pathways involved in programmed cell death, potentially reducing unnecessary cell loss due to radiation-induced apoptosis.
- **Regulation of Gene Expression**: It may influence the expression of genes related to stress responses, repair mechanisms, and cell survival.

Scientific Evidence and Research Findings

In Vitro Studies

- **Cell Culture Experiments**: Studies using cultured mammalian cells have demonstrated that pre-treatment with DMSO can enhance cell survival following ionizing radiation exposure.
  - *Example*: DMSO at concentrations of 1–2% (v/v) provided significant protection to human lymphocyte cultures against gamma radiation-induced chromosomal aberrations.
- **Mechanistic Insights**: Research indicates that DMSO's protective effects are dose-dependent and correlate with its free radical scavenging capacity.

In Vivo Studies

- **Animal Models**: Preclinical studies in rodents have explored DMSO's radioprotective effects when administered prior to radiation exposure.
  - *Example*: Mice pre-treated with DMSO showed increased survival rates and reduced tissue damage following lethal doses of whole-body irradiation.
- **Dose Optimization**: Effective radioprotection in animal models was observed with specific dosing regimens, highlighting the importance of timing and dosage in achieving protective effects.

Limitations of Current Research

- **Species Differences**: The extent of DMSO's radioprotective effects may vary between species, and results from animal studies may not directly translate to humans.

- **Concentration-Dependent Effects**: High concentrations required for radioprotection may not be clinically feasible due to potential toxicity.

- **Lack of Clinical Trials**: There is a scarcity of human clinical data assessing DMSO's efficacy as a radioprotective agent.

Potential Applications

Medical Radiation Exposure

- **Radiation Therapy**: DMSO could potentially protect normal tissues from collateral damage during radiotherapy for cancer treatment, thereby reducing side effects.

- **Diagnostic Imaging**: In procedures involving radiation exposure, such as CT scans or fluoroscopy, DMSO might offer protective benefits if administered appropriately.

Occupational and Environmental Exposure

- **Radiation Workers**: Individuals working in environments with radiation exposure may benefit from prophylactic use of radioprotective agents like DMSO.

- **Nuclear Accidents**: In the event of nuclear incidents, DMSO could be considered as part of emergency measures to mitigate radiation-induced harm.

Space Exploration

- **Astronaut Protection**: Space radiation poses significant risks to astronauts; DMSO may be investigated as a component of protective strategies against cosmic radiation.

Safety and Toxicity Considerations

Dosage and Administration

- **Therapeutic Window**: The effective radioprotective dose of DMSO must be balanced against its potential toxicity; high systemic doses may cause adverse effects.

- **Route of Administration**: Oral, intravenous, or topical administration routes have different pharmacokinetics and safety profiles that need careful evaluation.

Adverse Effects

- **Systemic Toxicity**: High doses of DMSO can lead to side effects such as headache, dizziness, nausea, and gastrointestinal disturbances.

- **Organ Toxicity**: Potential hepatotoxicity and nephrotoxicity may occur with excessive or prolonged use.

- **Allergic Reactions**: Hypersensitivity reactions, although rare, can present significant risks.

Interactions with Radiation Therapy

- **Tumor Protection Risk**: There is a concern that DMSO might also protect cancer cells during radiation therapy, potentially reducing treatment efficacy.

- **Timing of Administration**: Careful scheduling is necessary to maximize protection of normal tissues while not interfering with the intended cytotoxic effects on tumor cells.

Practical Considerations

Clinical Use and Medical Supervision

- **Lack of Regulatory Approval**: DMSO is not approved by regulatory agencies for use as a radioprotective agent in humans.

- **Medical Oversight**: Any consideration of DMSO for radiation protection should be under strict medical supervision within the context of clinical research.

- **Informed Consent**: Patients must be fully informed about the experimental nature of DMSO use for radiation protection, including potential risks and benefits.

Research and Development

- **Clinical Trials**: Well-designed clinical trials are necessary to evaluate the safety, optimal dosing, and efficacy of DMSO in radiation protection for humans.

- **Combination Therapies**: Investigating DMSO in combination with other radioprotective agents may enhance protective effects and reduce required dosages.

DMSO and Ionizing Radiation

Introduction

Ionizing radiation refers to high-energy particles or electromagnetic waves that have sufficient energy to ionize atoms or molecules by detaching electrons. Common sources include gamma rays, X-rays, alpha particles, beta particles, and neutrons. Exposure to ionizing radiation can cause significant biological damage, primarily through the generation of reactive oxygen species (ROS) and free radicals, leading to DNA damage, lipid peroxidation, and protein oxidation. Understanding and mitigating the harmful effects of ionizing radiation is crucial in fields such as radiation therapy, nuclear energy, and space exploration.

Dimethyl sulfoxide (DMSO) has been studied for its potential to modulate the effects of ionizing radiation on biological systems. This section delves into the specific interactions between DMSO and ionizing radiation, highlighting experimental evidence, proposed mechanisms unique to this context, and considerations for practical applications.

Mechanisms of Interaction Between DMSO and Ionizing Radiation

Radical Scavenging Specificity

While DMSO is known for its general antioxidant properties, its interaction with ionizing radiation involves specific radical scavenging activities:

- **Hydroxyl Radical Scavenging**: Ionizing radiation in aqueous environments primarily generates hydroxyl radicals (•OH), among the most reactive and damaging ROS. DMSO reacts with hydroxyl radicals to form methyl radicals and other less harmful species, thereby reducing immediate oxidative damage to biomolecules.

- **Formation of Protective Metabolites**: The reaction between DMSO and hydroxyl radicals produces methane sulfinic acid, which itself may possess radioprotective properties, contributing to a secondary line of defense against oxidative stress.

DNA Protection Mechanisms

DMSO's interaction with ionizing radiation extends to specific protective effects on DNA:

- **Prevention of Indirect DNA Damage**: Ionizing radiation causes DNA damage both directly and indirectly through water radiolysis, generating ROS that attack DNA. DMSO mitigates indirect damage by scavenging ROS before they interact with DNA.

- **Influence on DNA Repair Pathways**: Some studies suggest that DMSO may modulate the activity of DNA repair enzymes, enhancing the cell's ability to correct radiation-induced lesions, though the exact mechanisms remain under investigation.

Modulation of Radiation-Induced Signal Transduction

Ionizing radiation activates various cellular signaling pathways related to stress responses, apoptosis, and survival:

- **Alteration of Signal Transduction Cascades**: DMSO may influence key signaling molecules such as p53, ATM (ataxia-telangiectasia mutated), and NF-κB (nuclear factor kappa-light-chain-enhancer of activated B cells), potentially altering the cellular response to DNA damage.

- **Impact on Cell Cycle Checkpoints**: By affecting the regulation of cell cycle checkpoints, DMSO might reduce the propagation of damaged cells, contributing to genomic stability post-radiation.

Experimental Evidence

Studies on Cellular Models

Research utilizing various cellular models has provided insights into DMSO's effects under ionizing radiation:

- **Human Lymphocyte Cultures**: DMSO pre-treatment in human lymphocytes exposed to gamma radiation resulted in a significant decrease in micronuclei formation, indicating reduced chromosomal damage.
- **Cancer Cell Lines**: Investigations using tumor cell lines revealed that DMSO can differentially affect cancer cells and normal cells under radiation, sometimes enhancing radiosensitivity in cancer cells while protecting normal cells, though results are context-dependent.

Animal Studies

In vivo experiments have explored DMSO's potential radioprotective effects in whole organisms:

- **Mouse Models**: Mice administered DMSO before exposure to lethal doses of gamma radiation exhibited increased survival rates and reduced hematopoietic system damage. Hematological parameters such as white blood cell counts recovered more rapidly in DMSO-treated groups.
- **Dose-Response Relationships**: Studies have emphasized the importance of DMSO concentration, with optimal protective effects observed at specific doses. Excessive doses did not confer additional benefits and could introduce toxicity.

Type-Specific Radiation Effects

Research indicates that DMSO's protective efficacy may vary with different types of ionizing radiation:

- **Gamma Rays and X-Rays**: DMSO has shown significant protective effects against low linear energy transfer (LET) radiation like gamma rays and X-rays due to the predominance of hydroxyl radical formation.
- **Neutron and Heavy Ion Radiation**: Protection against high LET radiation such as neutron or heavy ion exposure is less pronounced, possibly because damage from these types is more direct and less mediated by free radicals that DMSO can scavenge.

Applications in Radiobiology and Medicine

Radioprotective Agent in Medical Settings

- **Bone Marrow Transplantation**: DMSO is used as a cryoprotectant for hematopoietic stem cells, and its potential to protect these cells from radiation-induced damage during transplantation procedures has been explored.
- **Adjunct in Radiation Therapy**: There's ongoing research into using DMSO to shield normal tissues during radiotherapy. Careful consideration is required to avoid protecting cancer cells, which could reduce treatment efficacy.

Space Radiation Protection

- **Astronaut Health**: With increased interest in long-duration space missions, DMSO's potential to mitigate cosmic radiation effects on astronauts is a subject of investigation, focusing on preserving neural and ocular function.

Limitations and Challenges

Selectivity and Specificity

- **Cancer Cell Protection Risk**: A significant concern is DMSO's non-selective protection, which might extend to malignant cells, potentially diminishing the effectiveness of radiotherapy.
- **Variable Efficacy**: The degree of protection offered by DMSO can vary widely depending on cell type, radiation dose, and environmental conditions, complicating its application.

Toxicity and Side Effects

- **Concentration-Dependent Toxicity**: Protective concentrations of DMSO in vitro may not be achievable in vivo without causing adverse effects, such as neurotoxicity or organ dysfunction.

- **Metabolic Impacts**: High doses of DMSO might interfere with cellular metabolism and function independent of radiation exposure, necessitating careful dosing strategies.

Usage Before Medical Imaging and Air Travel

Introduction

Exposure to ionizing radiation is a concern in certain everyday situations, notably during medical imaging procedures and air travel. Medical imaging techniques such as X-rays and computed tomography (CT) scans involve low doses of radiation, which, while minimal, can accumulate with repeated exposure. Similarly, passengers and crew on high-altitude flights are subject to increased levels of cosmic radiation compared to ground-level exposure. The potential use of dimethyl sulfoxide (DMSO) as a radioprotective agent in these contexts has garnered interest due to its antioxidant properties. This section examines the theoretical basis, current evidence, safety considerations, and practical implications of using DMSO before medical imaging and air travel.

Radiation Exposure in Medical Imaging and Air Travel

Medical Imaging Procedures

- **Diagnostic Imaging**: X-rays and CT scans are invaluable diagnostic tools that use ionizing radiation to create images of internal body structures. While the radiation doses are generally low, concerns arise with cumulative exposure, especially in patients requiring frequent imaging.

- **Radiation Dose Estimates**: A standard chest X-ray delivers approximately 0.1 millisieverts (mSv), whereas a CT scan of the abdomen can deliver up to 10 mSv. For perspective, the average annual background radiation exposure is about 3 mSv.

Air Travel Radiation Exposure

- **Cosmic Radiation**: At high altitudes, the atmosphere is thinner, providing less shielding from cosmic rays. This results in higher radiation exposure for airline passengers and crew compared to ground level.

- **Dose Estimates**: A typical transatlantic flight exposes an individual to about 0.03–0.05 mSv. While this is low, frequent flyers and aircrew may accumulate higher doses over time.

Theoretical Basis for DMSO Use

Antioxidant Properties of DMSO

- **Free Radical Scavenging**: DMSO is known for its ability to scavenge free radicals, particularly hydroxyl radicals generated during ionizing radiation exposure. This property suggests a potential to mitigate radiation-induced oxidative damage.

Potential Radioprotective Mechanisms

- **DNA Protection**: By neutralizing reactive species, DMSO may reduce indirect DNA damage caused by radiation-induced free radicals.

- **Cellular Defense Enhancement**: DMSO might bolster cellular antioxidant defenses, potentially preserving cell integrity during low-dose radiation exposure.

Current Evidence and Research Findings

Preclinical Studies

- **In Vitro Experiments**: Laboratory studies have demonstrated that DMSO can protect cultured cells from high-dose radiation-induced damage. However, these studies often involve radiation levels significantly higher than those encountered during medical imaging or air travel.

Lack of Clinical Evidence

- **Human Studies**: There is a paucity of clinical research evaluating DMSO's efficacy as a radioprotective agent in humans exposed to low-dose radiation typical of medical imaging or air travel.

- **Dose Discrepancy**: The protective effects observed in preclinical studies typically require DMSO concentrations or doses that are not practical or safe for routine human use in these contexts.

Regulatory Status

- **Not Approved for Radioprotection**: DMSO is not approved by regulatory agencies for use as a radioprotective agent in medical imaging or air travel scenarios.

Safety and Practical Considerations

Potential Risks of DMSO Use

- **Adverse Effects**: Topical or systemic administration of DMSO can cause side effects such as skin irritation, garlic-like body odor, headache, dizziness, and gastrointestinal disturbances.

- **Systemic Toxicity**: Unsupervised use, especially at high doses, may lead to organ toxicity, including hepatotoxicity and nephrotoxicity.

Medical Supervision Necessity

- **Professional Guidance**: Any consideration of DMSO use should be under the supervision of a qualified healthcare professional to evaluate potential risks and benefits.

- **Lack of Dosage Guidelines**: There are no established dosing regimens for DMSO as a radioprotective agent in these settings, increasing the risk of improper use.

Alternative Protective Measures

- **Minimizing Unnecessary Exposure**: Adhering to medical guidelines that recommend imaging studies only when necessary reduces cumulative radiation exposure.

- **Protective Shielding**: In medical imaging, the use of lead aprons and other shielding devices effectively minimizes radiation exposure to non-targeted body areas.

- **Radiation Monitoring**: For frequent flyers and aircrew, monitoring radiation doses and adhering to occupational exposure limits is advisable.

Recommendations and Guidelines

Current Medical Guidelines

- **No Endorsement of DMSO Use**: Medical authorities do not recommend the use of DMSO as a radioprotective agent before medical imaging or air travel due to insufficient evidence of efficacy and safety concerns.

- **Evidence-Based Practices**: Emphasis is placed on evidence-based strategies for radiation protection, such as optimizing imaging protocols to use the lowest effective radiation dose.

Consultation with Healthcare Providers

- **Individual Risk Assessment**: Individuals concerned about radiation exposure should discuss their specific situation with healthcare professionals.

- **Medical Advice**: Decisions regarding the use of any supplement or medication for radiation protection should be based on medical advice and current scientific evidence.

Chapter 5: Recipes and Formulations

Preparing DMSO Solutions for Different Concentrations

Introduction

Dimethyl sulfoxide (DMSO) is a highly polar organic solvent with the unique ability to dissolve both polar and nonpolar compounds. Its versatility makes it valuable in various fields, including pharmaceuticals, biotechnology, and chemical research. Preparing DMSO solutions of precise concentrations is essential for experimental reproducibility, accurate dosing, and safety compliance. This section outlines the methodologies for preparing DMSO solutions at different concentrations, emphasizing best practices, calculations, and safety precautions.

Properties Relevant to Solution Preparation

Before delving into the preparation methods, it is crucial to understand certain properties of DMSO that influence solution formulation:

- **Molecular Weight**: DMSO has a molecular weight of 78.13 g/mol.

- **Density**: The density of pure DMSO at 25°C is approximately 1.100 g/mL.

- **Miscibility**: DMSO is miscible with water and a wide range of organic solvents.

- **Hygroscopic Nature**: DMSO is hygroscopic and can absorb moisture from the air, potentially altering concentration if not properly handled.

General Considerations

- **Purity of DMSO**: Use high-purity, pharmaceutical-grade or analytical-grade DMSO to ensure consistency and minimize impurities that could affect experimental outcomes.

- **Solvent Compatibility**: Verify the compatibility of DMSO with other solvents or solutes to prevent precipitation or chemical reactions.

- **Temperature Control**: Perform preparations at room temperature unless specific protocols require otherwise, as temperature fluctuations can affect volume and concentration.

- **Equipment Calibration**: Use calibrated pipettes, volumetric flasks, and balances for accurate measurements.

Materials and Equipment

- **DMSO**: High-purity solvent appropriate for the intended application.

- **Solvent or Diluent**: Distilled water or other solvents as required.

- **Volumetric Flasks**: Class A flasks of appropriate volume (e.g., 10 mL, 25 mL, 50 mL, 100 mL).

- **Pipettes and Pipettors**: For precise measurement of liquids.

- **Analytical Balance**: For weighing solids when preparing solutions by weight.

- **Personal Protective Equipment (PPE)**: Gloves, lab coat, safety goggles.

- **Stirring Equipment**: Magnetic stirrer or vortex mixer to ensure homogeneity.

- **Storage Containers**: Chemically compatible containers with airtight seals.

Molar Solutions

To prepare molar solutions:

- Moles of DMSO=Desired Molarity (mol/L)×Final Volume (L)\
- Mass of DMSO (g)=Moles of DMSO×Molecular Weight of DMSO (g/mol)

Step-by-Step Procedures

Preparing a Specific % v/v DMSO Solution

Example: Prepare 100 mL of a 10% v/v DMSO solution.

1. **Calculate the Volume of DMSO Needed**:

$$Volume\ of\ DMSO = \left(\frac{10\%}{100\%}\right) x\ 100\ mL = 10\ mL$$

2. **Measure the DMSO**:

   o   Using a calibrated pipette, measure 10 mL of DMSO.

   o   Transfer the DMSO to a 100 mL volumetric flask.

3. **Add Diluent**:

   o   Add distilled water or the specified solvent to the flask containing DMSO.

   o   Fill the flask to the calibration mark with the diluent, ensuring the bottom of the meniscus aligns with the mark.

4. **Mix Thoroughly**:

   o   Cap the flask and invert several times or use a magnetic stirrer to achieve a homogeneous solution.

5. **Label the Solution**:

   o   Indicate the concentration, solvent used, preparation date, and any safety warnings.

Preparing a Molar DMSO Solution

Example: Prepare 50 mL of a 1 M DMSO solution.

1. **Calculate the Moles of DMSO Needed**:

   Moles of DMSO=1 mol/L×0.050 L=0.050 mol

2. **Calculate the Mass of DMSO Needed**:

   Mass of DMSO=0.050 mol×78.13 g/mol=3.9065 g

3. **Weigh the DMSO**:

   o   Tare a container on an analytical balance.

   o   Accurately weigh 3.9065 g of DMSO.

4. **Dissolve and Dilute**:

   o   Transfer the DMSO to a 50 mL volumetric flask.

   o   Add an appropriate solvent (e.g., distilled water) to dissolve the DMSO.

   o   Fill the flask to the 50 mL mark with the solvent.

5. **Mix and Label**:

   o   Ensure complete dissolution and homogeneity.

   o   Label the solution with concentration, solvent, and preparation details.

Preparing Diluted Solutions from a Stock Solution

Example: Prepare 25 mL of a 5% v/v DMSO solution from a 25% v/v stock solution.

1. **Use the Dilution Formula**:

$$C_1V_1 = C_2V_2$$

Where:

- C1 = Concentration of stock solution (25% v/v)
- V1 = Volume of stock solution needed
- C2 = Desired concentration (5% v/v)
- V2 = Final volume of diluted solution (25 mL)

2. **Calculate the Volume of Stock Solution Needed**:

$$V_1 = \left(\frac{C_2 V_2}{C_1}\right) = \left(\frac{5\% \; x \; 25 \; mL}{25\%}\right) = 5 \; mL$$

3. **Measure and Mix**:
   - Measure 5 mL of the 25% stock solution.
   - Transfer to a 25 mL volumetric flask.
   - Add diluent up to the 25 mL mark.
   - Mix thoroughly.

4. **Label Appropriately**.

Safety Precautions

- **Personal Protective Equipment**: Always wear gloves, safety goggles, and lab coats when handling DMSO, as it can facilitate the transdermal absorption of contaminants.

- **Ventilation**: Work in a well-ventilated area or fume hood to avoid inhalation of vapors.

- **Handling and Storage**: Keep DMSO and its solutions in tightly sealed containers to prevent moisture absorption and degradation.

- **Spill Management**: In case of spills, clean immediately with appropriate absorbent materials and dispose of waste according to institutional guidelines.

Tips for Accurate Preparation

- **Temperature Equilibration**: Allow solvents and DMSO to reach room temperature to minimize volume variations due to thermal expansion.

- **Avoiding Contamination**: Use clean, dry equipment, and avoid touching pipette tips or flask rims.

- **Verification**: If critical, verify the concentration of the prepared solution using analytical techniques like refractometry or spectrophotometry.

Storage and Stability

- **Short-Term Storage**: Store DMSO solutions at room temperature if they will be used within a few days.

- **Long-Term Storage**: For extended storage, keep solutions at low temperatures (e.g., 4°C) to prevent microbial growth and chemical degradation.

- **Light Sensitivity**: Some solutes may be light-sensitive; protect solutions from light by using amber glassware or wrapping containers in aluminum foil.

Disposal Considerations

- **Chemical Waste**: Dispose of unused DMSO solutions and waste according to local regulations and institutional policies.

- **Environmental Impact**: DMSO is considered relatively non-toxic to the environment but should still be disposed of responsibly to prevent contamination.

Combining DMSO with Natural Remedies

Introduction

The integration of Dimethyl sulfoxide (DMSO) with natural remedies represents a burgeoning area of interest in complementary and alternative medicine. Natural remedies, encompassing herbal extracts, essential oils, vitamins, and other bioactive compounds, are widely utilized for their therapeutic benefits and minimal side effects. Combining DMSO with these natural agents aims to harness synergistic effects, enhancing therapeutic efficacy while potentially mitigating adverse reactions. This section explores the scientific rationale for such combinations, examines specific natural remedies commonly paired with DMSO, reviews existing research on their interactions, and discusses safety considerations and best practices for their application.

Scientific Rationale for Combining DMSO with Natural Remedies

Synergistic Enhancement of Therapeutic Effects

Combining DMSO with natural remedies can lead to synergistic interactions where the combined effect exceeds the sum of individual effects. This synergy can amplify therapeutic outcomes in areas such as wound healing, pain management, and inflammation reduction.

Improved Bioavailability and Penetration

DMSO's renowned ability to enhance the transdermal delivery of various compounds makes it an effective carrier for natural remedies that otherwise have limited absorption when applied topically. This improved bioavailability ensures that higher concentrations of active ingredients reach target tissues, enhancing their efficacy.

Multifaceted Mechanisms of Action

Natural remedies often possess diverse biological activities, such as antimicrobial, anti-inflammatory, and antioxidant properties. When combined with DMSO, these multifaceted mechanisms can provide comprehensive therapeutic benefits, addressing multiple aspects of a condition simultaneously.

Common Natural Remedies Combined with DMSO

Aloe Vera

Properties: Aloe vera is renowned for its soothing, moisturizing, and wound-healing properties. It contains bioactive compounds like polysaccharides, vitamins, and enzymes that promote tissue repair and reduce inflammation.

Combination with DMSO: When combined with DMSO, aloe vera gel can penetrate deeper into the skin, enhancing its moisturizing and healing effects. This combination is particularly beneficial in treating burns, abrasions, and other skin injuries.

Turmeric (Curcumin)

Properties: Turmeric contains curcumin, a potent anti-inflammatory and antioxidant compound. Curcumin has been studied for its role in mitigating oxidative stress and modulating inflammatory pathways.

Combination with DMSO: DMSO can enhance the absorption of curcumin through the skin, potentially increasing its anti-inflammatory and analgesic effects. This combination may be effective in managing chronic inflammatory conditions such as arthritis.

Arnica Montana

Properties: Arnica is widely used for its anti-inflammatory and analgesic properties, particularly in the treatment of bruises, sprains, and muscle soreness. It contains sesquiterpene lactones and flavonoids that contribute to its therapeutic effects.

Combination with DMSO: When used together, DMSO facilitates the deeper penetration of arnica's active compounds, enhancing its efficacy in reducing pain and swelling associated with soft tissue injuries.

Essential Oils (e.g., Lavender, Tea Tree)

Properties: Essential oils like lavender and tea tree possess antimicrobial, anti-inflammatory, and soothing properties. Lavender oil is often used for its calming effects, while tea tree oil is valued for its antiseptic qualities.

Combination with DMSO: DMSO can act as a carrier for essential oils, improving their penetration and stability on the skin. This combination can be effective in treating minor infections, reducing inflammation, and providing analgesic benefits.

Vitamin E

Properties: Vitamin E is a powerful antioxidant that protects cells from oxidative damage and promotes skin health. It is commonly used in skincare for its moisturizing and healing properties.

Combination with DMSO: The application of DMSO with vitamin E can enhance the antioxidant protection of the skin, aiding in the repair of damaged tissues and preventing oxidative stress-related skin aging.

Research Evidence on DMSO and Natural Remedy Combinations

Preclinical Studies

- **Wound Healing**: In vitro studies have demonstrated that the combination of DMSO and aloe vera accelerates fibroblast proliferation and collagen synthesis more effectively than either agent alone, suggesting enhanced wound closure and tissue regeneration.

- **Inflammation**: Animal models of arthritis treated with both DMSO and curcumin showed a more significant reduction in joint inflammation and pain compared to treatment with either compound alone, indicating a synergistic anti-inflammatory effect.

Clinical Studies

- **Topical Treatments**: Clinical trials involving patients with musculoskeletal injuries have reported improved pain relief and reduced swelling when DMSO was used in conjunction with arnica gel, compared to placebo or arnica alone.

- **Skin Conditions**: Studies on burn patients have found that DMSO combined with aloe vera reduces healing time and minimizes scarring more effectively than standard treatments, highlighting the potential benefits of this combination in dermatological applications.

Limitations of Current Research

- **Sample Sizes**: Many studies investigating the combination of DMSO with natural remedies involve small participant numbers, limiting the generalizability of the findings.

- **Methodological Variability**: Differences in concentrations, application methods, and outcome measures across studies hinder the ability to draw definitive conclusions about the efficacy of these combinations.

- **Lack of Long-Term Data**: There is a scarcity of long-term studies assessing the sustained benefits and safety of combined DMSO and natural remedy treatments.

Safety Considerations

Potential Risks and Adverse Effects

- **Skin Irritation**: Both DMSO and certain natural remedies can cause skin irritation, redness, or allergic reactions. When combined, the risk may increase, necessitating cautious application and monitoring.

- **Transdermal Absorption**: DMSO's ability to enhance the penetration of other compounds means that natural remedies administered with DMSO can enter the systemic circulation more readily. This increased absorption may lead to unintended side effects, especially with potent natural agents.

- **Sensitivity and Allergies**: Individuals may be sensitive or allergic to specific natural remedies, and combining them with DMSO could exacerbate these reactions. Patch testing is recommended before widespread application.

Best Practices for Safe Combination

- **Patch Testing**: Conduct a patch test on a small area of skin to assess tolerance before applying the combination to larger or more sensitive areas.

- **Gradual Introduction**: Start with lower concentrations of both DMSO and the natural remedy to evaluate the skin's response, gradually increasing as tolerated.

- **Professional Guidance**: Consult with healthcare professionals, especially when dealing with chronic or severe conditions, to ensure appropriate usage and to avoid interactions with other treatments.

Contraindications

- **Pregnancy and Lactation**: Both DMSO and certain natural remedies may have contraindications during pregnancy and breastfeeding. It is essential to seek medical advice before use in these populations.

- **Pre-existing Medical Conditions**: Individuals with underlying health issues, such as liver or kidney disease, should exercise caution and consult healthcare providers before using DMSO in combination with natural remedies.

Practical Application Guidelines

Formulation and Preparation

- **Optimal Concentrations**: Determine the appropriate concentrations of DMSO and the natural remedy based on the specific condition and patient tolerance. Commonly, DMSO concentrations range from 10% to 70%, while natural remedies are used as per standard topical formulations.

- **Homogeneous Mixing**: Ensure thorough mixing of DMSO and natural remedies to achieve a consistent and effective solution. Utilize appropriate mixing techniques such as magnetic stirring or vortexing.

Application Techniques

- **Topical Application**: Apply the combined solution evenly over the affected area, ensuring full coverage without excessive pooling, which could increase the risk of irritation.

- **Frequency of Use**: Adhere to recommended application frequencies, typically two to three times daily, adjusting based on individual response and tolerance.

Storage and Stability

- **Proper Storage**: Store combined DMSO and natural remedy formulations in airtight containers, away from direct sunlight and extreme temperatures to maintain stability and prevent degradation.

- **Shelf Life**: Be aware of the shelf life of both DMSO and the natural remedy, ensuring that preparations are used within their effective periods to guarantee efficacy and safety.

Future Research Directions

Comprehensive Clinical Trials

- **Efficacy Assessment**: Large-scale, randomized controlled trials are needed to evaluate the therapeutic benefits and safety of combining DMSO with various natural remedies across different conditions.

- **Standardized Protocols**: Developing standardized protocols for dosing, application methods, and outcome measurements will enhance the comparability and reliability of future studies.

Mechanistic Studies

- **Understanding Synergy**: Investigate the molecular and cellular mechanisms underlying the synergistic effects of DMSO and natural remedies to optimize combinations for specific therapeutic outcomes.

- **Biomarker Identification**: Identify biomarkers that predict positive responses to combined treatments, facilitating personalized medicine approaches.

Development of Advanced Formulations

- **Enhanced Delivery Systems**: Explore advanced drug delivery systems, such as liposomes or nanoparticles, to further improve the stability and targeted delivery of combined DMSO and natural remedy formulations.

- **Sustained-Release Mechanisms**: Develop formulations that provide sustained release of active compounds, reducing the frequency of application and enhancing patient compliance.

Essential Oil Blends

Introduction

Essential oils are volatile, aromatic compounds extracted from plants, renowned for their therapeutic properties, including antimicrobial, anti-inflammatory, analgesic, and mood-enhancing effects. When integrated with Dimethyl sulfoxide (DMSO), a potent solvent and carrier agent, the efficacy of essential oils can be significantly enhanced. This synergy leverages DMSO's ability to facilitate deeper penetration of essential oils into tissues, thereby amplifying their biological activities. This section delves into the formulation of essential oil blends with DMSO, elucidates their mechanisms of action, reviews scientific evidence supporting their combined use, and outlines safety protocols and best practices for their application.

Mechanisms of Action in Essential Oil and DMSO Blends

Enhanced Transdermal Delivery

- **Solvent Properties of DMSO**: DMSO's high polarity allows it to disrupt the lipid matrix of the stratum corneum, enhancing the permeation of essential oil constituents into deeper layers of the skin and underlying tissues.

- **Increased Bioavailability**: By facilitating the transport of essential oils across biological membranes, DMSO increases the bioavailability of active compounds, ensuring higher concentrations reach target sites for therapeutic action.

Synergistic Biological Activities

- **Amplified Anti-Inflammatory Effects**: Essential oils such as lavender and chamomile possess intrinsic anti-inflammatory properties. When combined with DMSO, which also modulates inflammatory pathways, the resultant blend can provide a more robust reduction in inflammation.

- **Complementary Antimicrobial Actions**: Essential oils like tea tree and eucalyptus are known for their antimicrobial efficacy. DMSO can enhance the penetration of these oils into microbial cells, potentially increasing their bactericidal and fungicidal effects.

Neuroprotective and Analgesic Synergy

- **Pain Modulation**: Essential oils such as peppermint and rosemary have analgesic properties. DMSO's ability to stabilize neuronal membranes and modulate ion channels can complement these effects, offering enhanced pain relief.

- **Mood Enhancement**: Aromatic compounds from essential oils can influence neurotransmitter levels and mood states. DMSO's interaction with neural pathways may potentiate these psychological benefits, providing a holistic approach to pain and stress management.

Common Essential Oil Blends with DMSO

Lavender and Tea Tree Oil Blend

Components:

- **Lavender Oil**: Known for its calming, anti-inflammatory, and analgesic properties.

- **Tea Tree Oil**: Renowned for its potent antimicrobial and anti-inflammatory effects.

- **DMSO**: Acts as a carrier to enhance the penetration and efficacy of the essential oils.

Applications:

- **Wound Care**: This blend can be applied to minor cuts, abrasions, and burns to promote healing, reduce inflammation, and prevent infection.

- **Skin Infections**: Effective in managing fungal and bacterial skin infections due to the enhanced antimicrobial activity.

Peppermint and Eucalyptus Oil Blend

Components:

- **Peppermint Oil**: Contains menthol, which provides cooling and analgesic effects.

- **Eucalyptus Oil**: Offers anti-inflammatory and decongestant properties.

- **DMSO**: Facilitates deeper penetration for more effective relief.

Applications:

- **Muscle Pain Relief**: Ideal for treating muscle strains, sprains, and tension headaches by providing rapid analgesia and reducing muscle inflammation.

- **Respiratory Support**: Can be used for topical application to relieve sinus congestion and improve breathing by enhancing the penetration of eucalyptus's decongestant properties.

Rosemary and Frankincense Oil Blend

Components:

- **Rosemary Oil**: Exhibits anti-inflammatory, analgesic, and cognitive-enhancing effects.

- **Frankincense Oil**: Known for its anti-inflammatory, immune-modulating, and skin-rejuvenating properties.

- **DMSO**: Enhances the absorption and efficacy of both essential oils.

Applications:

- **Joint Pain Management**: Effective in alleviating symptoms of arthritis and other joint-related conditions by reducing inflammation and pain.

- **Skin Rejuvenation**: Promotes skin healing and reduces the appearance of scars and wrinkles through enhanced delivery of regenerative compounds.

Scientific Evidence Supporting DMSO and Essential Oil Blends

Preclinical Studies

- **Anti-Inflammatory Synergy**: In vitro studies have shown that blends of DMSO with essential oils like lavender and tea tree exhibit greater inhibition of pro-inflammatory cytokines (e.g., IL-6, TNF-α) compared to individual components.

- **Antimicrobial Efficacy**: Research indicates that DMSO-enhanced essential oil blends possess superior antimicrobial activity against common pathogens such as *Staphylococcus aureus* and *Candida albicans*.

Clinical Studies

- **Wound Healing**: Clinical trials involving patients with minor wounds demonstrated that DMSO and lavender oil blends accelerated healing times and reduced infection rates more effectively than standard treatments.

- **Pain Management**: Patients with chronic musculoskeletal pain reported significant pain reduction and improved mobility when using peppermint and eucalyptus oil blends with DMSO compared to placebo applications.

Mechanistic Insights

- **Cellular Uptake**: Studies suggest that DMSO increases the cellular uptake of essential oil constituents, enhancing their intracellular concentrations and therapeutic actions.

- **Gene Expression Modulation**: Combined treatments have been observed to influence the expression of genes related to inflammation, oxidative stress, and cell survival, contributing to their enhanced therapeutic effects.

Safety Considerations and Best Practices

Potential Risks and Adverse Effects

- **Skin Irritation and Sensitization**: Both DMSO and essential oils can cause skin irritation, redness, or allergic reactions, especially at higher concentrations. Combining them may increase the risk, necessitating cautious application.

- **Systemic Absorption**: DMSO's ability to enhance transdermal absorption means that essential oil constituents can enter the systemic circulation more readily, potentially leading to systemic side effects.

Best Practices for Safe Combination

- **Patch Testing**: Conduct a patch test on a small skin area to assess tolerance and identify any allergic reactions before widespread application.

- **Concentration Management**: Use appropriate concentrations of both DMSO and essential oils to balance efficacy with safety. Typically, DMSO concentrations range from 10% to 70%, while essential oils are used in low dilutions (e.g., 1-5%) to minimize irritation.

- **Gradual Introduction**: Introduce the blend gradually, starting with lower concentrations and increasing as tolerated to monitor for adverse reactions.

Regulatory and Quality Assurance

- **Quality of Ingredients**: Utilize high-purity, pharmaceutical-grade DMSO and essential oils to ensure consistency, potency, and minimize the presence of contaminants.

- **Compliance with Guidelines**: Adhere to regulatory guidelines and institutional protocols regarding the preparation, storage, and application of DMSO and essential oil blends.

Practical Application Guidelines

Formulation Techniques

- **Homogeneous Mixing**: Ensure thorough blending of DMSO with essential oils using appropriate mixing techniques such as magnetic stirring or vortexing to achieve a uniform solution.

- **Sterile Preparation**: Prepare blends in a clean environment to prevent contamination, especially when intended for wound care or sensitive skin applications.

Application Methods

- **Topical Application**: Apply the essential oil and DMSO blend evenly over the affected area using clean hands or applicators. Avoid excessive amounts to reduce the risk of irritation.

- **Massage Therapy**: Incorporate the blend into massage oils to enhance deep tissue penetration and provide therapeutic benefits during manual therapy sessions.

Storage and Stability

- **Proper Storage**: Store essential oil and DMSO blends in airtight, opaque containers to protect them from light, moisture, and air, which can degrade active compounds.

- **Shelf Life Management**: Use prepared blends within a specified timeframe, typically within one to two weeks, to ensure potency and reduce the risk of microbial growth.

Herbal Extracts

Introduction

Herbal extracts have been integral to traditional medicine systems worldwide, offering a diverse array of bioactive compounds with therapeutic potential. These extracts, derived from various parts of plants, including leaves, roots, flowers, and bark, possess properties such as antioxidant, anti-inflammatory, antimicrobial, and immunomodulatory effects. Combining Dimethyl sulfoxide (DMSO) with herbal extracts aims to enhance the efficacy and bioavailability of these natural agents through DMSO's solvent and carrier capabilities. This section explores the scientific foundation for integrating DMSO with herbal extracts, highlights specific herbal combinations, reviews supporting research, and discusses safety considerations and best practices for their application.

Scientific Rationale for Combining DMSO with Herbal Extracts

Enhanced Solubility and Bioavailability

- **Solvent Properties of DMSO**: DMSO's ability to dissolve both polar and nonpolar compounds allows it to effectively solubilize a wide range of herbal extract constituents, ensuring uniform distribution and consistent dosing.

- **Increased Absorption**: DMSO facilitates the permeation of herbal compounds across biological membranes, enhancing their systemic absorption and therapeutic reach.

Synergistic Pharmacological Effects

- **Complementary Mechanisms**: Herbal extracts often contain multiple active compounds that work synergistically. When combined with DMSO, these compounds can interact more effectively with cellular targets, amplifying their overall pharmacological effects.

- **Multi-Target Modulation**: The combination allows for simultaneous modulation of various biological pathways, providing a comprehensive approach to managing complex health conditions.

Common Herbal Extracts Combined with DMSO

Turmeric (Curcuma longa)

Properties: Turmeric contains curcumin, a compound renowned for its potent anti-inflammatory and antioxidant properties. Curcumin has been extensively studied for its role in mitigating chronic inflammation and oxidative stress-related diseases.

Combination with DMSO: DMSO enhances the solubility and skin penetration of curcumin, facilitating its deeper absorption into tissues. This combination is particularly effective in managing inflammatory skin conditions and musculoskeletal pain.

Applications:

- **Arthritis Relief**: Reduces joint inflammation and pain through enhanced delivery of curcumin to affected areas.

- **Skin Conditions**: Assists in the treatment of psoriasis and eczema by delivering curcumin more effectively to inflamed skin regions.

Ginger (Zingiber officinale)

Properties: Ginger contains bioactive compounds such as gingerol and shogaol, which exhibit anti-inflammatory, analgesic, and digestive properties. These compounds help alleviate nausea, reduce muscle pain, and manage inflammatory responses.

Combination with DMSO: DMSO improves the bioavailability of ginger's active constituents, allowing for more effective systemic and topical applications.

Applications:

- **Nausea Management**: Enhances the antiemetic effects of ginger when used in formulations for motion sickness or chemotherapy-induced nausea.

- **Muscle Pain Relief**: Facilitates deeper penetration of ginger extracts for more effective alleviation of muscle soreness and stiffness.

Arnica Montana

Properties: Arnica is traditionally used for its anti-inflammatory and analgesic effects, particularly in treating bruises, sprains, and muscle soreness. It contains sesquiterpene lactones and flavonoids that contribute to its therapeutic actions.

Combination with DMSO: DMSO acts as a carrier, enhancing the absorption of arnica's active compounds into the skin and underlying tissues.

Applications:

- **Sports Injuries**: Accelerates recovery from sprains and strains by delivering arnica more effectively to injured areas.

- **Bruise Reduction**: Enhances the anti-inflammatory effects of arnica, promoting faster resolution of bruising.

Milk Thistle (Silybum marianum)

Properties: Milk thistle contains silymarin, a complex of flavonolignans known for their hepatoprotective and antioxidant properties. Silymarin aids in liver detoxification and protects against oxidative damage.

Combination with DMSO: DMSO enhances the bioavailability of silymarin, potentially increasing its protective effects on liver tissues.

Applications:

- **Liver Support**: Improves the efficacy of milk thistle in supporting liver function and protecting against toxins.

- **Antioxidant Therapy**: Facilitates the delivery of silymarin to tissues requiring oxidative stress mitigation.

Scientific Evidence Supporting DMSO and Herbal Extract Combinations

Preclinical Studies

- **Anti-Inflammatory Synergy**: In vitro studies have demonstrated that DMSO combined with curcumin significantly reduces the expression of pro-inflammatory cytokines (e.g., IL-6, TNF-α) more effectively than either agent alone.

- **Enhanced Antioxidant Activity**: Animal models treated with DMSO and ginger extracts showed greater reduction in oxidative stress markers compared to single treatments, indicating enhanced antioxidant protection.

Clinical Studies

- **Arthritis Management**: Clinical trials involving patients with rheumatoid arthritis reported that topical formulations containing DMSO and arnica resulted in greater pain relief and reduced joint swelling compared to arnica alone.

- **Skin Healing**: Studies on burn patients found that DMSO-enhanced turmeric formulations accelerated epithelialization and reduced scar formation more effectively than standard treatments.

Mechanistic Insights

- **Cellular Uptake**: Research indicates that DMSO increases the cellular uptake of herbal compounds, leading to higher intracellular concentrations and more pronounced biological effects.

- **Gene Expression Modulation**: Combined treatments with DMSO and herbal extracts have been shown to influence the expression of genes involved in inflammation, apoptosis, and cellular repair mechanisms, thereby enhancing therapeutic outcomes.

Safety Considerations and Best Practices

Potential Risks and Adverse Effects

- **Skin Irritation**: Both DMSO and certain herbal extracts can cause skin irritation, redness, or allergic reactions. The combination may heighten these risks, particularly at higher concentrations.

- **Systemic Absorption**: DMSO's ability to enhance transdermal absorption means that herbal compounds can enter systemic circulation more readily, potentially leading to systemic side effects.

- **Interactions with Medications**: Herbal extracts may interact with pharmaceuticals, and DMSO can alter the pharmacokinetics of co-administered drugs. This necessitates careful consideration of potential drug-herb interactions.

Best Practices for Safe Combination

- **Patch Testing**: Conduct a patch test on a small area of skin to assess tolerance and identify any allergic reactions before widespread application.

- **Controlled Concentrations**: Use appropriate concentrations of DMSO and herbal extracts to balance efficacy with safety. Typically, DMSO concentrations range from 10% to 70%, while herbal extracts are used in standardized dilutions as per recommended guidelines.

- **Gradual Introduction**: Introduce the combination gradually, starting with lower concentrations and increasing as tolerated to monitor for adverse reactions.

- **Professional Oversight**: Consult healthcare professionals, especially when treating chronic or severe conditions, to ensure appropriate usage and avoid adverse interactions.

Contraindications

- **Pregnancy and Lactation**: Both DMSO and certain herbal extracts may have contraindications during pregnancy and breastfeeding. Use should be avoided unless deemed necessary by a healthcare provider.

- **Pre-existing Medical Conditions**: Individuals with liver or kidney dysfunction, skin disorders, or other chronic health issues should exercise caution and seek medical advice before using combined DMSO and herbal extract treatments.

Practical Application Guidelines

Formulation Techniques

- **Accurate Measurement**: Utilize calibrated pipettes, syringes, and volumetric flasks to ensure precise measurements of DMSO and herbal extracts.

- **Homogeneous Mixing**: Employ thorough mixing techniques, such as magnetic stirring or vortexing, to achieve a uniform solution and ensure consistent therapeutic effects.

- **Sterile Conditions**: Prepare formulations in a clean environment to prevent contamination, especially when intended for wound care or sensitive skin applications.

Application Methods

- **Topical Application**: Apply the DMSO and herbal extract blend evenly over the affected area using clean hands or sterile applicators. Avoid excessive amounts to minimize the risk of irritation.

- **Massage Therapy**: Incorporate the blend into massage oils to enhance deep tissue penetration and provide therapeutic benefits during manual therapy sessions.

Storage and Stability

- **Proper Storage**: Store combined DMSO and herbal extract formulations in airtight, opaque containers to protect them from light, moisture, and air, which can degrade active compounds.

- **Shelf Life Management**: Use prepared blends within a specified timeframe, typically within one to two weeks, to ensure potency and reduce the risk of microbial growth.

Disposal Considerations

- **Chemical Waste**: Dispose of unused DMSO and herbal extract solutions according to local regulations and institutional policies to prevent environmental contamination.

- **Environmental Impact**: While DMSO is considered relatively non-toxic to the environment, responsible disposal practices should be followed to minimize ecological impact.

DMSO Gel and Cream Preparations

Introduction

Dimethyl sulfoxide (DMSO) is widely utilized in topical formulations such as gels and creams due to its exceptional solvent properties and ability to enhance the transdermal delivery of active compounds. These formulations offer a convenient and effective means of administering DMSO for various therapeutic applications, including pain management, inflammation reduction, and enhanced delivery of co-administered drugs or natural remedies. This section provides a comprehensive guide to preparing DMSO-based gels and creams, detailing essential ingredients, preparation methods, concentration guidelines, stability considerations, and safety protocols to ensure effective and safe formulations.

Properties of DMSO Relevant to Gel and Cream Preparations

Understanding the physicochemical properties of DMSO is crucial for successful formulation development:

- **Solvent Capability**: DMSO's ability to dissolve both polar and nonpolar substances makes it an excellent carrier for a wide range of active ingredients.

- **Viscosity**: Pure DMSO has a relatively low viscosity, which can be adjusted in gel and cream formulations to achieve desired textures and application characteristics.

- **Skin Penetration**: DMSO enhances the permeability of the stratum corneum, facilitating deeper penetration of active compounds into target tissues.

- **Stability**: DMSO is chemically stable under normal storage conditions but can absorb moisture from the environment, potentially affecting formulation consistency.

Essential Ingredients for DMSO Gels and Creams

Successful gel and cream formulations require a combination of DMSO with other components to achieve optimal texture, stability, and efficacy:

- **DMSO**: The primary active solvent, typically used in concentrations ranging from 10% to 70% depending on the application and desired penetration depth.

- **Gelling Agents**: Substances such as carbomers, hydroxyethyl cellulose, or xanthan gum are used to provide viscosity and structure to gel formulations.

- **Emollients**: Ingredients like glycerin, propylene glycol, or natural oils (e.g., jojoba oil, coconut oil) enhance skin hydration and suppleness in cream formulations.

- **Emulsifiers**: Necessary for cream formulations to maintain a stable mixture of oil and water phases. Examples include cetyl alcohol, stearyl alcohol, and polysorbates.

- **Preservatives**: To prevent microbial growth and extend shelf life, preservatives such as parabens, phenoxyethanol, or benzyl alcohol are incorporated.

- **Active Ingredients**: Optional compounds like essential oils, herbal extracts, or pharmaceutical agents that benefit from enhanced delivery via DMSO.

- **pH Adjusters**: Agents like triethanolamine or sodium hydroxide are used to adjust the pH of the formulation to match skin's natural pH and ensure stability of the gelling agent.

Step-by-Step Preparation Protocols

Preparing a DMSO Gel

Example: Preparation of a 50% v/v DMSO Gel using Carbomer as a gelling agent.

Ingredients:

- 50 mL DMSO
- 1 g Carbomer 940
- 5 mL Triethanolamine (TEA)
- 20 mL Distilled Water
- 2 g Glycerin
- 0.5 g Preservative (e.g., phenoxyethanol)
- Optional: 1-2 mL essential oil for fragrance or additional therapeutic effects

Procedure:

1. **Hydration of Carbomer**:

   o In a clean, sterilized mixing container, add 1 g Carbomer 940 to 20 mL of distilled water.

   o Stir gently using a magnetic stirrer to disperse the Carbomer completely, allowing it to hydrate and swell. This process may take several minutes.

2. **Addition of Glycerin**:

   o Incorporate 2 g glycerin into the hydrated Carbomer solution, mixing thoroughly to ensure uniform distribution.

3. **Neutralization**:

   o Gradually add 5 mL of triethanolamine (TEA) to the mixture while continuously stirring. TEA neutralizes the Carbomer, transforming the solution into a clear, gel-like consistency.

4. **Incorporation of DMSO**:

   o Slowly add 50 mL of DMSO to the gel base, stirring continuously to achieve a homogeneous mixture. Ensure that the DMSO is added in increments to prevent separation.

5. **Preservative and Optional Ingredients**:

   o Add 0.5 g of preservative to the mixture, ensuring it is evenly distributed.

   o If desired, incorporate 1-2 mL of essential oil for fragrance or additional therapeutic benefits, stirring thoroughly.

6. **Final Mixing**:

   o Use a magnetic stirrer or homogenizer to ensure complete blending of all components, resulting in a smooth, consistent gel.

7. **Packaging and Labeling**:

   o Transfer the prepared gel into sterile, airtight containers.

   o Label the containers with concentration details, ingredients, preparation date, and any safety warnings.

Preparing a DMSO Cream

Example: Preparation of a 30% v/v DMSO Cream using cetyl alcohol as an emulsifier.

Ingredients:

- 30 mL DMSO

- 15 g Cetyl Alcohol

- 20 g Stearyl Alcohol

- 40 g Distilled Water

- 10 g Glycerin

- 2 g Emulsifying Wax (e.g., polysorbate 60)

- 0.5 g Preservative (e.g., benzyl alcohol)

- Optional: 1-2 mL herbal extract or essential oil

Procedure:

1. **Oil Phase Preparation**:

   o In a heat-resistant container, combine 15 g cetyl alcohol, 15 g stearyl alcohol, and 2 g emulsifying wax.

- Heat the mixture gently in a water bath until all components are fully melted and homogeneous, typically around 70-75°C.

2. **Water Phase Preparation**:

    - In a separate container, combine 40 g distilled water and 10 g glycerin.

    - Heat the water phase to the same temperature as the oil phase to ensure proper emulsification.

3. **Emulsification**:

    - Slowly pour the hot oil phase into the water phase while continuously stirring with a magnetic stirrer or homogenizer.

    - Maintain stirring until the mixture begins to emulsify and thicken, forming a creamy consistency.

4. **Cooling and Incorporation of DMSO**:

    - Allow the mixture to cool to below 40°C while stirring gently to prevent separation.

    - Gradually add 30 mL of DMSO to the cooling cream base, stirring continuously to ensure even distribution.

5. **Addition of Preservative and Optional Ingredients**:

    - Incorporate 0.5 g of preservative into the mixture, ensuring thorough blending.

    - If desired, add 1-2 mL of herbal extract or essential oil, stirring well to achieve a uniform cream.

6. **Final Mixing**:

    - Continue stirring until the cream reaches room temperature and achieves a smooth, homogenous texture.

7. **Packaging and Labeling**:

    - Transfer the prepared cream into sterilized, airtight containers.

    - Label the containers with concentration details, ingredients, preparation date, and any safety warnings.

Concentration Considerations

- **Therapeutic Goals**: The concentration of DMSO in gels and creams should align with the intended therapeutic application. Higher concentrations (up to 70%) are typically used for deep tissue penetration and enhanced delivery of active ingredients, while lower concentrations (10-30%) are suitable for mild applications and minimizing irritation.

- **Patient Tolerance**: Individual sensitivity to DMSO varies. It is advisable to start with lower concentrations and gradually increase as tolerated, especially in sensitive populations such as children, elderly individuals, or those with compromised skin integrity.

- **Regulatory Guidelines**: Adhere to local regulatory standards regarding maximum allowable concentrations of DMSO in topical formulations to ensure compliance and safety.

Stability and Storage

- **Homogeneity**: Ensure thorough mixing during preparation to maintain a consistent distribution of DMSO and other ingredients, preventing phase separation over time.

- **Shelf Life**: Properly prepared gels and creams can be stable for several months when stored under optimal conditions. Regularly inspect formulations for signs of separation, discoloration, or microbial contamination.

- **Storage Conditions**: Store formulations in a cool, dark place away from direct sunlight and extreme temperatures to preserve the integrity of DMSO and other active components.

- **Preservative Efficacy**: Adequate preservative concentrations are essential to prevent microbial growth, especially in aqueous-based formulations.

Safety Protocols

- **Personal Protective Equipment (PPE)**: Wear gloves, safety goggles, and protective clothing when handling DMSO and preparing formulations to prevent accidental skin absorption and exposure.

- **Ventilation**: Conduct preparation in a well-ventilated area or fume hood to minimize inhalation of DMSO vapors, which can cause respiratory irritation.

- **Handling Precautions**: Avoid contact with eyes and mucous membranes. In case of accidental exposure, rinse thoroughly with water and seek medical attention if irritation persists.

- **Labeling and Documentation**: Clearly label all formulations with concentration details, ingredients, preparation date, and safety warnings. Maintain documentation of batch preparations for quality control and traceability.

Quality Control Measures

- **Consistency Checks**: Regularly assess the viscosity, homogeneity, and pH of prepared gels and creams to ensure consistency across batches.

- **Microbial Testing**: Implement routine microbial testing, especially for aqueous-based formulations, to verify the effectiveness of preservatives and prevent contamination.

- **Batch Testing**: For pharmaceutical-grade preparations, conduct batch testing for potency, purity, and stability as per regulatory requirements.

Troubleshooting Common Issues

- **Phase Separation**: Occurs when ingredients are not adequately mixed or when incompatible components are used. To resolve, gently reheat the formulation and stir vigorously to re-emulsify.

- **Clumping or Grittiness**: Indicates incomplete dissolution of gelling agents or improper mixing. Ensure thorough hydration and use appropriate mixing techniques to achieve a smooth texture.

- **Excessive Viscosity**: May result from over-gelling or high concentrations of gelling agents. Adjust the amount of gelling agent or incorporate thinning agents such as glycerin or propylene glycol.

- **Color and Odor Changes**: Could signify degradation or contamination. Inspect raw materials for quality and ensure proper storage conditions to prevent such changes.

Applications of DMSO Gels and Creams

- **Pain Management**: Topical gels and creams with DMSO are used to alleviate localized pain from conditions such as arthritis, muscle strains, and joint inflammation by enhancing the delivery of analgesic agents.

- **Inflammation Reduction**: Formulations designed to reduce inflammation can incorporate anti-inflammatory herbs or pharmaceutical agents, benefiting from DMSO's penetration-enhancing properties.

- **Wound Healing**: DMSO-based gels and creams can promote faster wound healing by facilitating the delivery of growth factors, antimicrobial agents, and soothing compounds.

- **Transdermal Drug Delivery**: These formulations serve as effective carriers for various medications, improving their bioavailability and therapeutic efficacy when applied topically.

- **Cosmetic Applications**: Enhanced delivery of anti-aging compounds, vitamins, and skin-rejuvenating agents in cosmetic formulations can be achieved through DMSO gels and creams.

Internal Use Recipes

Introduction

Dimethyl sulfoxide (DMSO) is a versatile solvent known for its ability to penetrate biological membranes, facilitating the delivery of various therapeutic agents. While DMSO is commonly used topically, its internal administration has garnered interest for its potential systemic therapeutic benefits, including anti-inflammatory, analgesic, and antioxidant effects. However, internal use of DMSO requires meticulous preparation, precise dosing, and stringent safety measures due to its potent biological activity and potential side effects. This section provides scientifically grounded formulations for internal administration of DMSO, outlining preparation protocols, dosage guidelines, and critical safety considerations. It is imperative to underscore that these recipes are intended solely for informational purposes and should **only** be undertaken under the guidance and supervision of qualified healthcare professionals.

Safety and Regulatory Considerations

Before delving into specific recipes, it is crucial to acknowledge the following safety and regulatory aspects:

- **Medical Supervision**: Internal use of DMSO should always be conducted under the supervision of a healthcare provider to monitor efficacy and mitigate risks.

- **Regulatory Status**: DMSO is approved by the U.S. Food and Drug Administration (FDA) for specific indications, such as interstitial cystitis, but its internal use for other conditions remains off-label and should comply with local regulatory guidelines.

- **Potential Side Effects**: Internal DMSO can cause gastrointestinal disturbances, headaches, dizziness, and a distinctive garlic-like odor. Severe adverse effects may include liver or kidney toxicity at high doses.

- **Contraindications**: Individuals with liver or kidney impairment, pregnant or breastfeeding women, and those with known hypersensitivity to DMSO should avoid internal use.

Essential Ingredients and Equipment

- **Pharmaceutical-Grade DMSO**: Ensure the use of high-purity DMSO to minimize impurities and contaminants.

- **Distilled Water or Appropriate Solvents**: For diluting DMSO to desired concentrations.

- **Oral Syringes or Measuring Devices**: For accurate dosing.

- **Sterile Containers**: To store prepared solutions safely.

- **Personal Protective Equipment (PPE)**: Gloves and safety goggles to prevent accidental exposure.

Preparation Protocols

1. Oral DMSO Solution

Purpose: To deliver DMSO systemically for its anti-inflammatory and analgesic properties.

Concentration: 10% v/v DMSO solution

Ingredients:

- 10 mL pharmaceutical-grade DMSO

- 90 mL distilled water

Equipment:

- 100 mL sterile glass bottle

- Graduated cylinder

- Stirring rod or magnetic stirrer

Procedure:

1. **Sanitize Equipment**: Ensure all equipment and containers are sterile to prevent contamination.

2. **Measure DMSO**: Using a graduated cylinder, accurately measure 10 mL of pharmaceutical-grade DMSO.

3. **Dilute DMSO**: Pour the measured DMSO into a 100 mL sterile glass bottle.

4. **Add Distilled Water**: Add 90 mL of distilled water to the bottle, ensuring precise measurement to achieve a 10% concentration.

5. **Mix Thoroughly**: Use a stirring rod or magnetic stirrer to ensure complete homogenization of the solution.

6. **Label the Solution**: Clearly label the container with concentration, preparation date, and storage instructions.

7. **Storage**: Store the solution in a cool, dark place away from direct sunlight. Refrigeration is recommended to enhance stability.

Dosage Guidelines:

- **Initial Dose**: Start with a low dose, such as 1 mL (equivalent to 0.1 grams of DMSO), taken orally once daily.

- **Titration**: Gradually increase the dose under medical supervision based on patient response and tolerance, not exceeding 4 mL (0.4 grams of DMSO) per day.

Administration Instructions:

- **Oral Intake**: DMSO solution can be taken directly or mixed with a non-flavored beverage to mask the odor.

- **Frequency**: Typically administered once daily, preferably in the morning to monitor any immediate side effects.

2. Intravenous (IV) DMSO Solution

Purpose: To provide rapid systemic delivery of DMSO for acute inflammatory conditions or other specific medical indications.

Concentration: 70% v/v DMSO in saline solution

Ingredients:

- 70 mL pharmaceutical-grade DMSO

- 30 mL sterile saline solution (0.9% NaCl)

Equipment:

- Sterile IV bag (100 mL capacity)

- Syringes and needles for mixing

- Sterile gloves and aseptic technique tools

Procedure:

1. **Aseptic Environment**: Perform the preparation in a sterile environment, such as a laminar flow hood, to maintain sterility.

2. **Measure DMSO**: Using a sterile syringe, accurately measure 70 mL of pharmaceutical-grade DMSO.

3. **Dilute with Saline**: Add the 70 mL of DMSO to a sterile IV bag containing 30 mL of sterile saline solution.

4. **Mix Thoroughly**: Gently invert the IV bag multiple times to ensure thorough mixing without introducing air bubbles.

5. **Inspect for Clarity**: Ensure the solution is clear and free from particulates or precipitates.

6. **Label the Solution**: Clearly label the IV bag with concentration, preparation date, and expiration date.

7. **Storage**: Store the IV solution in a controlled environment, adhering to sterility and stability requirements.

Dosage Guidelines:

- **Standard Dose**: Administered by a healthcare professional, typically not exceeding 100 mL of 70% DMSO saline solution per dose.

- **Administration Rate**: Infuse slowly over a period of 30 minutes to 1 hour to monitor for adverse reactions.

A

118

dministration Instructions:

- **IV Infusion**: Administered intravenously through an existing IV line, with continuous monitoring for any signs of adverse effects.
- **Medical Supervision**: Must be performed by qualified healthcare personnel with emergency protocols in place.

3. DMSO Capsules

Purpose: To provide a convenient and controlled method for oral administration of DMSO.

Concentration: 50 mg DMSO per capsule

Ingredients:

- Pharmaceutical-grade DMSO
- Gelatin capsules (size appropriate for 50 mg dosage)
- Filling machine or manual capsule filling tools

Equipment:

- Capsule filling machine (optional)
- Digital scale for precise measurement
- Sterile workspace

Procedure:

1. **Sanitize Workspace**: Ensure all equipment and surfaces are clean and sterile.
2. **Measure DMSO**: Accurately weigh 50 mg of pharmaceutical-grade DMSO using a digital scale.
3. **Fill Capsules**:
   - **Manual Method**: Use a capsule filling tray to manually place DMSO into each gelatin capsule.
   - **Machine Method**: Utilize a capsule filling machine for higher efficiency and consistency.
4. **Seal Capsules**: Ensure each capsule is properly sealed to prevent leakage.
5. **Label the Capsules**: Clearly label the container with dosage information, concentration, and storage instructions.
6. **Storage**: Store capsules in a cool, dry place, away from direct sunlight and moisture.

Dosage Guidelines:

- **Initial Dose**: Start with one capsule (50 mg) taken orally once daily.
- **Titration**: Gradually increase the dose under medical supervision based on patient response, not exceeding five capsules (250 mg) per day.

Administration Instructions:

- **Oral Intake**: Swallow capsules whole with water, preferably with meals to minimize gastrointestinal discomfort.
- **Frequency**: Typically administered once daily, with potential increases based on therapeutic needs and tolerance.

Stability and Shelf Life

- **Oral Solutions**: Remain stable for up to six months when stored in airtight, opaque containers at room temperature. Refrigeration can extend shelf life.

- **IV Solutions**: Must be used within 24 hours of preparation to maintain sterility and prevent microbial growth.

- **Capsules**: Have a shelf life of up to one year when stored properly, protected from light and moisture.

Quality Control Measures

- **Concentration Verification**: Use analytical methods such as high-performance liquid chromatography (HPLC) to verify the concentration of DMSO in prepared solutions.

- **Sterility Testing**: Especially critical for IV solutions, ensure all preparations are free from microbial contamination through appropriate sterilization techniques.

- **pH Monitoring**: Check the pH of solutions to ensure they are within physiologically acceptable ranges, typically between 5.5 and 7.5 for oral and IV preparations.

Troubleshooting Common Issues

- **Precipitation**: Occurs when DMSO concentration exceeds solubility limits for certain solutes. Adjust concentrations or use compatible solvents to resolve.

- **Clarity Issues**: Cloudiness may indicate contamination or improper mixing. Re-mix the solution gently or prepare a fresh batch if contamination is suspected.

- **Capsule Leakage**: Ensure proper sealing of gelatin capsules and avoid overfilling to prevent leakage.

Disposal Considerations

- **Chemical Waste**: Dispose of unused DMSO solutions and capsules according to local hazardous waste regulations to prevent environmental contamination.

- **Contaminated Materials**: Treat all materials that have come into contact with DMSO as hazardous waste, following institutional and regulatory guidelines.

Juices and Beverages

Introduction

Dimethyl sulfoxide (DMSO) is recognized for its remarkable solvent properties and ability to penetrate biological membranes, facilitating the delivery of various therapeutic agents. While topical applications of DMSO are well-documented, its internal administration through juices and beverages is an emerging area of interest. This method aims to enhance the palatability and ease of consumption of DMSO, potentially broadening its therapeutic applications. However, internal use of DMSO requires careful formulation, precise dosing, and stringent safety measures due to its potent biological activity and potential side effects. This section provides scientifically grounded formulations for incorporating DMSO into juices and beverages, outlines dosage guidelines, reviews relevant research, and emphasizes critical safety considerations.

Scientific Rationale for Using Juices and Beverages

Enhanced Palatability and Compliance

- **Taste Masking**: DMSO possesses a strong garlic-like odor and bitter taste, which can be unpleasant when consumed alone. Incorporating DMSO into flavorful juices and beverages can significantly improve palatability, encouraging consistent use and enhancing patient compliance.

- **Ease of Administration**: Juices and beverages provide a convenient and familiar medium for ingestion, making it easier for individuals to incorporate DMSO into their daily routines without the need for specialized equipment or preparation.

Improved Bioavailability

- **Solubilization of Active Compounds**: Juices and beverages can effectively dissolve DMSO and other co-administered bioactive compounds, ensuring uniform distribution and consistent dosing.

- **Hydration Support**: Consuming DMSO with fluids supports proper hydration, which is essential for its systemic distribution and excretion, thereby enhancing its therapeutic efficacy.

Common Juices and Beverages for DMSO Administration

1. Citrus-Based DMSO Juice

Ingredients:

- 10 mL pharmaceutical-grade DMSO
- 90 mL freshly squeezed orange or grapefruit juice

Preparation:

1. **Sanitize Equipment**: Ensure all utensils and containers are clean to prevent contamination.
2. **Mix Ingredients**: In a sterile glass container, combine 10 mL of DMSO with 90 mL of citrus juice.
3. **Stir Well**: Use a sterile stirring rod or magnetic stirrer to ensure thorough mixing.
4. **Storage**: Store the mixture in a refrigerated, airtight container and use within 24 hours to prevent spoilage.

Usage:

- **Dosage**: Begin with a low dose, such as 1 mL of the DMSO juice, taken once daily under medical supervision.
- **Administration**: Consume the mixture directly or dilute further with water to mask the taste.

2. Herbal Tea Infusion with DMSO

Ingredients:

- 10 mL pharmaceutical-grade DMSO
- 200 mL brewed herbal tea (e.g., chamomile, peppermint)

Preparation:

1. **Brew Tea**: Prepare 200 mL of herbal tea according to package instructions.
2. **Cool the Tea**: Allow the tea to cool to room temperature to prevent degradation of DMSO.
3. **Combine DMSO**: Add 10 mL of DMSO to the brewed tea.
4. **Mix Thoroughly**: Stir the mixture until homogenous.
5. **Storage**: Store in a sealed container and consume within 12 hours.

Usage:

- **Dosage**: Administer 1 mL of the DMSO-infused herbal tea once daily, increasing the dose gradually as tolerated.

3. Smoothie Incorporation

Ingredients:

- 5 mL pharmaceutical-grade DMSO
- 100 mL fruit smoothie (e.g., banana, berries, spinach)
- 50 mL almond milk or other preferred base

Preparation:

1. **Prepare Smoothie**: Blend fruits and almond milk to create a smooth consistency.
2. **Add DMSO**: Incorporate 5 mL of DMSO into the smoothie mixture.
3. **Blend Again**: Ensure the DMSO is evenly distributed by blending the mixture for an additional 30 seconds.

4. **Storage**: Consume immediately or refrigerate for up to 24 hours.

Usage:

- **Dosage**: Start with 0.5 mL of the DMSO smoothie, taken once daily, increasing to a maximum of 2 mL as tolerated.

Scientific Evidence and Research Findings

Preclinical Studies

- **Animal Models**: Rodent studies have demonstrated that oral administration of DMSO can modulate inflammatory responses and provide neuroprotective effects. However, optimal dosing and long-term impacts require further exploration.

Clinical Studies

- **Limited Human Research**: Clinical trials specifically investigating DMSO ingestion via juices and beverages are scarce. Most existing data are anecdotal or derived from studies involving higher doses for specific conditions like interstitial cystitis.

Mechanistic Insights

- **Anti-Inflammatory Pathways**: DMSO interacts with inflammatory mediators, reducing the production of pro-inflammatory cytokines such as IL-6 and TNF-α, thereby contributing to its therapeutic effects.

- **Antioxidant Activity**: By scavenging free radicals, DMSO helps mitigate oxidative stress, which is implicated in various chronic diseases and inflammatory conditions.

Safety and Precautions

Potential Adverse Effects

- **Gastrointestinal Distress**: DMSO ingestion can cause nausea, diarrhea, and abdominal cramps, particularly at higher doses.

- **Garlic-Like Odor and Taste**: Due to its metabolism to dimethyl sulfide, DMSO can impart a garlic-like odor to breath and sweat, which may be socially uncomfortable.

- **Skin Irritation**: Oral intake of DMSO can lead to systemic absorption, potentially causing skin irritation or sensitization.

Contraindications

- **Pregnancy and Lactation**: DMSO is not recommended for pregnant or breastfeeding women due to limited safety data.

- **Liver and Kidney Impairment**: Patients with hepatic or renal dysfunction should avoid internal DMSO use, as these organs are critical for DMSO metabolism and excretion.

Drug Interactions

- **Enhanced Absorption of Other Medications**: DMSO can increase the bioavailability of concurrently administered drugs, potentially leading to unexpected pharmacological effects or toxicity.

- **Consultation with Healthcare Provider**: It is essential to inform healthcare providers about any concurrent medications or supplements to manage potential interactions.

Dosage Considerations

- **Start Low, Go Slow**: Initiate with the lowest possible dose to assess tolerance, gradually increasing based on therapeutic response and absence of adverse effects.

- **Maximum Recommended Dose**: Do not exceed 4 mL of DMSO per day without medical supervision, as higher doses increase the risk of toxicity.

Monitoring and Medical Supervision

- **Regular Monitoring**: Patients using internal DMSO should undergo periodic evaluations to monitor liver and kidney function, as well as overall health status.

- **Emergency Protocols**: Be aware of signs of overdose or severe adverse reactions, such as respiratory distress, severe skin reactions, or significant gastrointestinal symptoms, and seek immediate medical attention if they occur.

Practical Application Guidelines

Formulation Techniques

- **Accurate Measurement**: Utilize precise measuring devices, such as syringes or graduated cylinders, to ensure accurate dosing of DMSO in beverages.

- **Uniform Mixing**: Thoroughly mix DMSO with the chosen juice or beverage to achieve a homogenous solution, preventing localized high concentrations that could increase irritation risk.

Administration Tips

- **Taste Masking**: Combine DMSO with strongly flavored or sweet juices to mask its unpleasant taste and odor, enhancing patient compliance.

- **Consistent Scheduling**: Administer DMSO at the same time each day to maintain stable blood levels and maximize therapeutic effects.

Storage and Stability

- **Refrigeration**: Store prepared DMSO beverages in the refrigerator to prolong shelf life and prevent microbial growth.

- **Short-Term Use**: Consume prepared solutions within 24-48 hours to ensure freshness and prevent degradation.

Preparation Example

Example Recipe: Ginger-Lemon DMSO Elixir

Ingredients:

- 10 mL pharmaceutical-grade DMSO

- 100 mL fresh lemon juice

- 50 mL ginger juice (freshly pressed)

- 50 mL filtered water

- 1 tablespoon honey (optional, for sweetness)

Procedure:

1. **Sanitize Equipment**: Sterilize all mixing containers and utensils to maintain solution purity.

2. **Mix Juices**: In a large sterile container, combine 100 mL of lemon juice and 50 mL of ginger juice.

3. **Dilute DMSO**: Add 10 mL of DMSO to the juice mixture, stirring thoroughly to ensure complete integration.

4. **Add Water and Sweetener**: Incorporate 50 mL of filtered water and 1 tablespoon of honey, mixing until fully dissolved.

5. **Final Stirring**: Use a magnetic stirrer or shake vigorously to achieve a uniform solution.

6. **Label and Store**: Pour the elixir into a sterile, airtight bottle, label it with concentration and preparation date, and refrigerate.

Usage:

- **Dose**: Take 1-2 mL of the ginger-lemon DMSO elixir once daily, preferably in the morning with breakfast.

Supplement Synergy (e.g., Vitamin C, MSM)

Introduction

Combining Dimethyl sulfoxide (DMSO) with dietary supplements such as Vitamin C and methylsulfonylmethane (MSM) has emerged as a strategic approach to enhance therapeutic outcomes through synergistic interactions. These supplements, renowned for their individual health benefits, may work in concert with DMSO to amplify their efficacy, improve bioavailability, and support overall wellness. This section explores the scientific rationale behind supplement synergy with DMSO, examines specific combinations involving Vitamin C and MSM, reviews relevant research findings, and discusses safety considerations and best practices for their integrated use.

Scientific Rationale for Supplement Synergy with DMSO

Enhanced Bioavailability and Absorption

- **DMSO as a Carrier**: DMSO's exceptional solvent properties facilitate the dissolution and transport of various bioactive compounds across biological membranes. When combined with supplements like Vitamin C and MSM, DMSO can enhance their absorption into systemic circulation, ensuring higher bioavailability and more effective physiological action.

- **Improved Cellular Uptake**: DMSO penetrates cellular membranes efficiently, potentially increasing the intracellular concentrations of co-administered supplements. This heightened uptake can optimize the biological activities of these supplements at the cellular level.

Synergistic Antioxidant and Anti-Inflammatory Effects

- **Complementary Mechanisms**: Vitamin C and MSM possess distinct antioxidant and anti-inflammatory properties that can complement DMSO's own biological activities. The combination may provide a multifaceted approach to reducing oxidative stress and inflammation, which are underlying factors in various chronic conditions.

- **Enhanced Free Radical Scavenging**: Both DMSO and Vitamin C are potent free radical scavengers. Their combined use may result in a more comprehensive neutralization of reactive oxygen species (ROS), thereby protecting cells from oxidative damage more effectively than either agent alone.

Specific Supplement Combinations

Vitamin C and DMSO

Properties of Vitamin C:

- **Antioxidant Role**: Vitamin C (ascorbic acid) is a vital antioxidant that protects cells from oxidative stress by neutralizing free radicals.

- **Collagen Synthesis**: It is essential for the synthesis and maintenance of collagen, supporting skin integrity and wound healing.

- **Immune Function**: Vitamin C enhances immune responses, aiding in the prevention and management of infections.

Synergy with DMSO:

- **Enhanced Antioxidant Protection**: The combination of Vitamin C's antioxidant capacity with DMSO's free radical scavenging enhances overall cellular protection against oxidative stress.

- **Improved Collagen Formation**: DMSO's ability to penetrate tissues can facilitate the delivery of Vitamin C to collagen-rich areas, promoting more effective collagen synthesis and tissue repair.

- **Immune Modulation**: Together, DMSO and Vitamin C may synergistically support immune function, providing a more robust defense against pathogens.

Research Evidence:

- **In Vitro Studies**: Laboratory research indicates that combined administration of DMSO and Vitamin C results in superior antioxidant effects compared to individual treatments, offering enhanced protection against oxidative damage in cultured cells.

- **Clinical Observations**: Preliminary clinical reports suggest that patients receiving both DMSO and Vitamin C exhibit improved outcomes in conditions characterized by high oxidative stress and impaired collagen synthesis, such as chronic wounds and inflammatory diseases.

Methylsulfonylmethane (MSM) and DMSO

Properties of MSM:

- **Sulfur Source**: MSM is a naturally occurring sulfur compound that contributes to the synthesis of connective tissues, including cartilage, tendons, and ligaments.

- **Anti-Inflammatory Effects**: It reduces inflammation by inhibiting pro-inflammatory cytokines and mediators, thereby alleviating pain and swelling.

- **Antioxidant Properties**: MSM scavenges free radicals, protecting cells from oxidative damage and supporting overall cellular health.

Synergy with DMSO:

- **Enhanced Joint Health**: The combination of MSM's role in connective tissue synthesis with DMSO's penetration capabilities can lead to more effective delivery of MSM to joint tissues, potentially improving conditions like osteoarthritis and rheumatoid arthritis.

- **Amplified Anti-Inflammatory Action**: Both MSM and DMSO independently reduce inflammation. Their combined use may result in a more pronounced anti-inflammatory effect, providing greater relief from pain and swelling.

- **Improved Cellular Protection**: MSM's antioxidant properties complement DMSO's ability to neutralize free radicals, offering comprehensive protection against oxidative stress at the cellular level.

Research Evidence:

- **Animal Studies**: In rodent models of arthritis, the combined administration of MSM and DMSO has demonstrated superior reduction in joint inflammation and pain compared to either agent alone, highlighting their synergistic anti-inflammatory effects.

- **Human Trials**: Clinical studies involving patients with osteoarthritis have reported enhanced joint mobility and decreased pain scores when MSM is administered alongside DMSO, suggesting improved therapeutic outcomes through their combined use.

Safety Considerations and Best Practices

Potential Risks and Adverse Effects

- **Increased Absorption Risks**: DMSO's ability to enhance the absorption of supplements means that higher systemic concentrations of Vitamin C and MSM may be achieved, which could potentially lead to adverse effects if not properly monitored.

- **Gastrointestinal Distress**: High doses of Vitamin C can cause gastrointestinal issues such as diarrhea and stomach cramps. When combined with DMSO, the risk may be elevated, necessitating careful dose management.

- **Skin Irritation and Sensitization**: DMSO can cause skin irritation and sensitization, especially at higher concentrations. When used with supplements that have their own irritation potentials, such as MSM, the likelihood of adverse skin reactions may increase.

Best Practices for Safe Combination

- **Medical Supervision**: Always undertake the combination of DMSO with supplements like Vitamin C and MSM under the guidance of a qualified healthcare professional to ensure appropriate dosing and monitor for adverse effects.

- **Start with Low Doses**: Initiate treatment with lower doses of both DMSO and the supplement, gradually increasing based on tolerance and therapeutic response. This approach minimizes the risk of side effects and allows for adjustment based on individual patient needs.

- **Monitor for Adverse Reactions**: Regularly assess for signs of gastrointestinal distress, skin irritation, or other adverse effects. Immediate discontinuation of the combination therapy should be considered if severe reactions occur.

- **Quality of Ingredients**: Use high-purity, pharmaceutical-grade DMSO and standardized supplements to ensure consistency, potency, and minimize the presence of contaminants that could contribute to adverse reactions.

Contraindications

- **Pregnancy and Lactation**: The combined use of DMSO with Vitamin C or MSM is not recommended during pregnancy and lactation due to limited safety data and potential risks to the fetus or infant.

- **Pre-existing Medical Conditions**: Individuals with liver or kidney dysfunction, as well as those with a history of allergic reactions to DMSO or the supplements, should avoid this combination unless specifically advised by a healthcare provider.

Practical Application Guidelines

Formulation Techniques

- **Accurate Measurement**: Utilize precise measuring devices, such as graduated syringes or digital scales, to ensure accurate dosing of DMSO and supplements.

- **Homogeneous Mixing**: Thoroughly mix DMSO with supplements to achieve a uniform solution, preventing localized high concentrations that could increase the risk of irritation or adverse effects.

- **Storage Conditions**: Store combined formulations in airtight, opaque containers to protect from light, moisture, and air, which can degrade active compounds. Refrigeration may be necessary to maintain stability and prolong shelf life.

Administration Methods

- **Oral Solutions**: Incorporate DMSO and supplements into palatable beverages or juices to enhance ingestion and absorption. Ensure the solution is well-mixed and consumed promptly to prevent degradation.

- **Capsule Formulations**: Encapsulate precise doses of DMSO and supplements to facilitate controlled and convenient oral administration. Use gelatin or vegetarian capsules as appropriate, ensuring complete sealing to prevent leakage.

- **Adjunctive Therapies**: Integrate the combination into a broader therapeutic regimen that includes dietary modifications, physical therapy, and other pharmacological treatments as recommended by healthcare providers.

Chapter 6: DMSO for Animals

Uses in Veterinary Medicine

Introduction

Dimethyl sulfoxide (DMSO) has established itself as a valuable tool in veterinary medicine, offering a range of therapeutic benefits across various animal species. Its unique physicochemical properties enable DMSO to act as both a solvent and a bioactive agent, facilitating the delivery of medications and enhancing therapeutic outcomes. Veterinarians employ DMSO in the treatment of musculoskeletal injuries, dermatological conditions, inflammatory disorders, and as a cryoprotectant in reproductive technologies. This section explores the diverse applications of DMSO in veterinary practice, elucidates the underlying mechanisms tailored to animal physiology, reviews scientific evidence supporting its efficacy, discusses administration protocols, addresses safety considerations, and highlights areas for future research.

Therapeutic Applications of DMSO in Veterinary Medicine

Musculoskeletal Injuries

DMSO is widely utilized in equine and canine medicine for managing musculoskeletal injuries, including joint inflammation, tendonitis, and osteoarthritis. Its analgesic and anti-inflammatory properties help reduce pain and swelling, promoting faster recovery and improved mobility.

- **Equine Applications**: In horses, DMSO is often administered intravenously or topically to treat joint inflammation and tendon injuries. It is used in combination with other anti-inflammatory agents to enhance therapeutic effects and accelerate healing.

- **Canine Applications**: Dogs with arthritis or tendon injuries benefit from DMSO's ability to penetrate tissues and deliver anti-inflammatory compounds directly to affected areas, reducing discomfort and improving joint function.

Dermatological Conditions

DMSO's ability to enhance the penetration of topical medications makes it an effective treatment for various skin conditions in animals, such as dermatitis, allergic reactions, and wounds.

- **Topical Treatments**: Applied as a gel or cream, DMSO facilitates the delivery of corticosteroids, antibiotics, and herbal extracts, enhancing their efficacy in treating inflammatory skin diseases and promoting wound healing.

- **Wound Management**: DMSO helps maintain a moist wound environment, reduces infection risk, and accelerates tissue regeneration, making it valuable in managing surgical wounds, burns, and traumatic injuries.

Inflammatory Disorders

DMSO is employed to manage systemic inflammatory conditions in animals, including autoimmune diseases and chronic inflammatory states.

- **Autoimmune Diseases**: In conditions like rheumatoid arthritis and systemic lupus erythematosus, DMSO's immunomodulatory effects help reduce autoimmune-mediated tissue damage and inflammation.

- **Chronic Inflammation**: DMSO assists in mitigating chronic inflammatory responses, improving quality of life and functional outcomes in animals with persistent inflammatory conditions.

Cryopreservation in Reproductive Technologies

In livestock breeding and conservation programs, DMSO is a critical cryoprotectant used in the preservation of gametes and embryos.

- **Sperm Preservation**: DMSO protects sperm cells during the freezing and thawing processes, maintaining their viability and fertility for artificial insemination and other reproductive techniques.

- **Embryo Storage**: It aids in preserving embryo integrity, ensuring successful implantation and development post-thawing, which is essential for breeding programs and species conservation efforts.

Antimicrobial Applications

DMSO's tissue-penetrating capabilities enhance the delivery of antimicrobial agents, making it effective in treating bacterial and fungal infections.

- **Bacterial Infections**: When combined with antibiotics, DMSO improves their penetration into infected tissues, enhancing their bactericidal effects and reducing infection severity.

- **Fungal Infections**: Similarly, DMSO enhances the efficacy of antifungal agents, aiding in the treatment of dermatophytic infections and other fungal-related skin conditions.

Oncology Support

DMSO is sometimes integrated into treatment protocols for animals with certain types of cancer, aiming to improve the delivery and efficacy of chemotherapeutic agents.

- **Chemotherapy Enhancement**: DMSO can increase the solubility and bioavailability of chemotherapeutic drugs, ensuring more effective targeting of tumor cells while potentially reducing systemic side effects.

- **Pain and Inflammation Management**: It also helps manage cancer-related pain and inflammation, improving the overall quality of life for affected animals.

Mechanisms of Action in Veterinary Applications

Solvent and Carrier Properties

DMSO's exceptional solvent capabilities allow it to dissolve a wide range of therapeutic agents, facilitating their delivery into tissues. This enhances the bioavailability and efficacy of medications administered both topically and systemically.

Anti-Inflammatory and Analgesic Effects

DMSO exerts potent anti-inflammatory and analgesic effects by inhibiting the synthesis of pro-inflammatory cytokines and reducing the infiltration of inflammatory cells into tissues. This dual action helps alleviate pain and swelling associated with various conditions.

Immunomodulatory Actions

DMSO modulates immune responses by influencing the activity of immune cells and altering cytokine production. This helps manage autoimmune disorders and reduce chronic inflammation, contributing to better disease control and symptom management.

Cryoprotective Properties

In reproductive technologies, DMSO acts as a cryoprotectant by preventing ice crystal formation during the freezing process. This protects cellular structures, ensuring the viability and functionality of gametes and embryos post-thawing.

Scientific Evidence and Research Findings

Musculoskeletal and Inflammatory Conditions

Numerous studies have demonstrated the efficacy of DMSO in reducing inflammation and pain in musculoskeletal injuries. For example, research in equine medicine shows that intravenous DMSO administration significantly decreases joint inflammation and accelerates tendon healing. Similarly, canine studies indicate that topical DMSO formulations improve mobility and reduce pain in arthritic joints.

Dermatological Applications

Clinical trials in companion animals have validated the use of DMSO-enhanced topical treatments in managing dermatitis and promoting wound healing. These studies highlight the superior outcomes achieved with DMSO formulations compared to standard treatments alone.

Cryopreservation Efficacy

Extensive research in livestock breeding confirms DMSO's role in preserving sperm and embryos. Studies indicate high post-thaw viability rates and successful fertilization outcomes, underscoring its importance in reproductive technologies and genetic preservation.

Antimicrobial Synergy

In vitro and in vivo studies reveal that DMSO enhances the antimicrobial efficacy of antibiotics and antifungals. For instance, DMSO combined with specific antibiotics shows increased bacterial killing rates, suggesting its potential to combat resistant infections more effectively.

Oncology Support

While research is still emerging, preliminary studies suggest that DMSO can improve chemotherapeutic outcomes by enhancing drug delivery and reducing tumor-related inflammation. However, more comprehensive clinical trials are needed to fully establish its role in veterinary oncology.

Administration Protocols

Intravenous Administration

For systemic conditions, DMSO is administered intravenously, often diluted with saline and combined with other anti-inflammatory or analgesic agents. Dosages are carefully calculated based on the animal's weight and condition, with treatment regimens typically involving multiple doses over several days.

Topical Application

Topical DMSO is prepared as gels, creams, or solutions, applied directly to the affected area. Concentrations range from 10% to 70%, depending on the condition being treated. Applications are usually performed multiple times daily to maintain therapeutic levels and promote healing.

Oral Administration

Although less common, oral DMSO formulations are used for systemic conditions in small animals. These formulations must be carefully dosed to avoid gastrointestinal side effects, with administration protocols tailored to individual tolerance and therapeutic needs.

Cryopreservation Procedures

In reproductive technologies, DMSO is incorporated into cryoprotective solutions for sperm and embryos. The preparation involves precise concentration adjustments and controlled freezing protocols to ensure maximum cell viability and functionality upon thawing.

Safety Considerations

Species-Specific Sensitivities

Different animal species exhibit varying sensitivities to DMSO. Cats, for example, are more susceptible to adverse reactions, necessitating lower doses and cautious administration compared to dogs and horses.

Dosage and Toxicity

Accurate dosing is critical to prevent toxicity. Overdosage can lead to adverse effects such as neurological disturbances, renal impairment, and gastrointestinal distress. Veterinary guidelines recommend starting with the lowest effective dose and adjusting based on the animal's response.

Allergic Reactions

Some animals may develop hypersensitivity to DMSO, manifesting as skin irritation, itching, or systemic allergic reactions. Patch testing and gradual introduction are recommended to minimize the risk of severe allergic responses.

Drug Interactions

DMSO can interact with various medications, altering their pharmacokinetics and effects. Comprehensive medical histories and careful monitoring are essential when combining DMSO with other treatments to avoid adverse interactions.

Handling and Storage

Proper handling and storage of DMSO are essential to maintain its efficacy and safety. It should be stored in tightly sealed containers, away from incompatible substances and extreme temperatures. Use appropriate personal protective equipment (PPE) to prevent accidental exposure during formulation and administration.

Dosage and Application for Pets

Introduction

Administering Dimethyl sulfoxide (DMSO) to pets requires precise dosage calculations and appropriate application methods to ensure safety and efficacy. DMSO's unique properties as a solvent and its intrinsic anti-inflammatory, analgesic, and antimicrobial effects make it a valuable adjunct in veterinary therapeutics. However, the correct dosage and application protocols must be meticulously followed to mitigate potential adverse effects and optimize therapeutic outcomes. This section provides scientifically grounded guidelines for determining appropriate DMSO dosages and application techniques for various pets, including dogs, cats, and horses, while emphasizing safety considerations and the importance of veterinary supervision.

General Dosage Guidelines

Determining the Appropriate Dose

The dosage of DMSO for pets is typically based on body weight, the condition being treated, and the method of administration. Precise dosing is crucial to maximize therapeutic benefits while minimizing the risk of toxicity.

- **Dosage Calculation**: The standard dosage range for DMSO in veterinary medicine is generally between 0.5 to 2 grams per kilogram of body weight per day. However, this can vary based on specific conditions and veterinary recommendations.

$$\text{Dosage (g/day)} = \text{Body Weight (kg)} \times \text{Dosage per kg (g/kg)}$$

- **Adjustments**: Dosages may need to be adjusted for animals with compromised liver or kidney function, as these organs are involved in metabolizing and excreting DMSO.

Species-Specific Dosage

Different species metabolize and respond to DMSO differently, necessitating tailored dosage protocols.

Dogs

- **Typical Dose**: 0.5 to 1.0 g/kg/day.

- **Administration Routes**: Topical application is most common, often combined with other anti-inflammatory agents.

- **Conditions Treated**: Arthritis, tendonitis, dermatitis, and wounds.

Cats

- **Typical Dose**: 0.25 to 0.5 g/kg/day.

- **Administration Routes**: Primarily topical due to cats' sensitivity to certain substances and potential for adverse reactions.

- **Conditions Treated**: Skin infections, minor wounds, and inflammatory conditions.

Horses

- **Typical Dose**: 1.0 to 2.0 g/kg/day.

- **Administration Routes**: Both intravenous (IV) and topical applications are utilized, depending on the condition.

- **Conditions Treated**: Joint inflammation, tendon injuries, and inflammatory diseases.

Application Methods

Topical Application

Topical application is the most common method for administering DMSO to pets due to its direct action on localized areas and minimal systemic absorption compared to other routes.

- **Formulations**: DMSO is typically prepared as gels, creams, or solutions. Concentrations range from 10% to 70%, with higher concentrations used for more severe conditions.

- **Procedure**:

  1. **Clean the Area**: Thoroughly clean and dry the affected area to remove dirt and debris, ensuring better absorption of DMSO.

  2. **Apply DMSO**: Using gloves, apply a thin layer of the DMSO formulation to the affected area.

  3. **Massage Gently**: Gently massage the area to facilitate penetration. Avoid excessive pressure to prevent skin irritation.

  4. **Cover if Necessary**: In some cases, covering the area with a bandage can enhance absorption and prevent the pet from licking the treated area.

Intravenous (IV) Administration

IV administration is employed primarily in larger animals like horses for systemic conditions where rapid and widespread distribution of DMSO is required.

- **Procedure**:

  1. **Prepare the Solution**: Dilute pharmaceutical-grade DMSO in sterile saline or another appropriate IV fluid, typically at a concentration of 10-20%.

  2. **Sterile Technique**: Use aseptic techniques to prevent contamination during preparation and administration.

  3. **Infusion Rate**: Administer the solution slowly over 30 minutes to 1 hour, monitoring the animal for any adverse reactions.

  4. **Post-Administration Monitoring**: Observe the animal for signs of discomfort, allergic reactions, or other side effects.

Oral Administration

Oral administration is less common and generally reserved for specific therapeutic protocols under strict veterinary supervision due to the strong taste and potential for gastrointestinal irritation.

- **Formulations**: DMSO can be mixed with palatable liquids like juices or encapsulated for easier ingestion.

- **Procedure**:

  1. **Measure the Dose**: Accurately measure the prescribed amount of DMSO.

  2. **Mix Thoroughly**: Combine DMSO with the chosen liquid to mask its taste.

  3. **Administer**: Offer the mixture to the pet using a syringe or a dropper, ensuring complete consumption.

  4. **Monitor**: Watch for any signs of gastrointestinal distress or adverse reactions.

Frequency and Duration

Frequency of Administration

- **Topical Treatments**: Typically applied 2-3 times daily, depending on the severity of the condition and the pet's tolerance.

- **IV Administration**: Generally administered once daily or as prescribed by a veterinarian, especially in acute conditions.

- **Oral Administration**: Administered once daily, with dosages potentially divided to reduce gastrointestinal irritation.

Duration of Treatment

- **Acute Conditions**: May require short-term use of DMSO, ranging from a few days to a couple of weeks, depending on the response.

- **Chronic Conditions**: Long-term administration may be necessary for managing chronic diseases like arthritis, with periodic reassessment by a veterinarian to adjust dosages and evaluate efficacy.

Safety Precautions

Monitoring and Adjustments

- **Regular Assessments**: Conduct regular veterinary check-ups to monitor the pet's response to DMSO therapy, adjusting dosages as needed based on therapeutic outcomes and any adverse effects.

- **Blood Work**: Periodic blood tests may be necessary to assess liver and kidney function, especially during prolonged DMSO therapy.

Adverse Effects Management

- **Skin Irritation**: If signs of irritation occur, reduce the concentration of DMSO or decrease the frequency of application. In severe cases, discontinue use and consult a veterinarian.

- **Gastrointestinal Issues**: For oral administration, if the pet experiences vomiting or diarrhea, reduce the dose or discontinue use and seek veterinary advice.

- **Allergic Reactions**: Immediate veterinary intervention is required if signs of an allergic reaction, such as swelling, difficulty breathing, or hives, are observed.

Contraindications

- **Pregnancy and Lactation**: DMSO is not recommended for pregnant or lactating animals due to limited safety data.

- **Pre-existing Conditions**: Animals with liver or kidney disease should avoid DMSO unless explicitly directed by a veterinarian, as these organs are critical for DMSO metabolism and excretion.

- **Drug Interactions**: DMSO can interact with certain medications, enhancing their absorption and effects. Comprehensive medical histories are essential to avoid adverse interactions.

Practical Tips for Effective Administration

- **Gradual Introduction**: Introduce DMSO gradually to allow the pet's system to acclimate, starting with lower doses and increasing as tolerated.

- **Consistent Routine**: Maintain a consistent administration schedule to ensure steady therapeutic levels and optimize treatment efficacy.

- **Proper Storage**: Store DMSO formulations in airtight, opaque containers away from direct sunlight and extreme temperatures to maintain stability and prevent degradation.

- **Hygiene Practices**: Use gloves when handling DMSO to prevent transdermal absorption of contaminants and to protect both the handler and the pet from potential irritation.

Chapter 7: Understanding Side Effects and Managing Risks

Common Side Effects (Skin Irritation, Odor)

Introduction

While Dimethyl sulfoxide (DMSO) is lauded for its versatile therapeutic applications, it is not devoid of side effects. Understanding the common adverse reactions associated with DMSO use is essential for both practitioners and users to ensure safe and effective therapy. This section delves into two of the most frequently reported side effects of DMSO: skin irritation and odor. It examines the underlying mechanisms, factors influencing their occurrence, strategies for mitigation, and clinical considerations to manage these side effects effectively.

Skin Irritation

Mechanisms of Skin Irritation

Skin irritation resulting from DMSO application primarily stems from its potent solvent properties. DMSO can disrupt the lipid bilayer of the stratum corneum, the outermost layer of the skin, increasing its permeability. While this characteristic enhances the transdermal delivery of therapeutic agents, it can also lead to:

- **Dermal Barrier Disruption**: By altering the lipid structure, DMSO compromises the skin's natural barrier, making it more susceptible to irritation and sensitivity.

- **Inflammatory Response**: The increased permeability can facilitate the penetration of other irritants or allergens present in the formulation, triggering an inflammatory response characterized by redness, itching, and swelling.

- **Cellular Stress**: High concentrations of DMSO may induce oxidative stress in keratinocytes, leading to cellular damage and inflammatory signaling.

Incidence and Severity

The incidence and severity of skin irritation vary based on several factors:

- **Concentration of DMSO**: Higher concentrations (above 50%) are more likely to cause significant irritation compared to lower concentrations (10-30%).

- **Duration of Exposure**: Prolonged contact with DMSO increases the risk of irritation. Extended application without breaks can exacerbate adverse skin reactions.

- **Individual Sensitivity**: Some individuals possess inherently more sensitive skin or pre-existing dermatological conditions, making them more prone to irritation.

- **Formulation Composition**: The presence of other active ingredients or excipients in the formulation can influence the extent of skin irritation. For instance, preservatives or fragrances may act as additional irritants.

Mitigation Strategies

Effective management of DMSO-induced skin irritation involves both preventive and responsive measures:

- **Gradual Introduction**: Begin with lower concentrations of DMSO and gradually increase as tolerated. This approach allows the skin to acclimate to DMSO's effects, reducing the likelihood of severe irritation.

- **Application Frequency**: Limit the frequency of application, especially during the initial stages of treatment. For example, applying DMSO once daily and increasing to twice daily based on tolerance can minimize adverse reactions.

- **Buffering Agents**: Incorporate buffering agents such as aloe vera or calendula extracts into DMSO formulations to soothe the skin and reduce irritation.

- **Protective Barriers**: Use emollients or occlusive dressings post-application to protect the skin from external irritants and maintain hydration, thereby enhancing barrier function.

- **pH Adjustment**: Formulate DMSO solutions at a pH compatible with skin physiology (typically between 5.5 and 7.0) to minimize irritation caused by pH imbalances.

- **Patch Testing**: Conduct patch tests on a small skin area prior to widespread application to assess individual sensitivity and prevent severe reactions.

Clinical Considerations

Healthcare providers should consider the following when addressing skin irritation caused by DMSO:

- **Patient Education**: Inform patients about the potential for skin irritation and the importance of adhering to recommended application protocols. Educate them on recognizing early signs of irritation and the steps to take if adverse reactions occur.

- **Monitoring and Follow-Up**: Schedule regular follow-ups to monitor skin health and adjust treatment regimens as necessary. Early intervention can prevent minor irritation from progressing to more severe dermatitis.

- **Alternative Formulations**: For patients who experience significant irritation, consider alternative formulations with lower DMSO concentrations or different delivery methods to balance efficacy with tolerability.

Odor

Mechanisms of Odor Formation

The characteristic garlic-like odor associated with DMSO use is primarily due to its metabolism into dimethyl sulfide (DMS), a volatile sulfur compound. This metabolic process occurs both systemically and at the site of application, leading to detectable odors emanating from breath, sweat, and urine.

- **Systemic Metabolism**: Once absorbed, DMSO is metabolized in the liver to DMS and other sulfur-containing compounds, which are then excreted via the respiratory and urinary systems.

- **Topical Metabolism**: Applied DMSO can also be metabolized locally in the skin, contributing to the odor through transdermal excretion.

Incidence and Impact

The odor associated with DMSO is universally experienced by users, regardless of the application method. While it is not harmful, it can be socially embarrassing and may affect adherence to therapy, especially in settings requiring close human interaction.

- **Concentration Correlation**: Higher concentrations of DMSO correlate with more pronounced odors due to increased production of DMS during metabolism.

- **Individual Metabolic Variability**: Differences in metabolic rates among individuals can influence the intensity and duration of the odor.

Mitigation Strategies

Several approaches can be employed to manage and reduce the impact of DMSO-induced odor:

- **Dosage Optimization**: Utilizing the lowest effective concentration of DMSO can minimize the production of DMS, thereby reducing odor intensity.

- **Application Timing**: Applying DMSO during times when the odor is less socially impactful (e.g., nighttime) can help manage its presence during peak social interactions.

- **Odor Masking Agents**: Incorporating fragrances or odor-neutralizing agents into DMSO formulations can help mask the garlic-like smell without interfering with therapeutic efficacy.

- **Hydration and Excretion**: Encouraging adequate hydration can facilitate the excretion of DMS and reduce the duration of detectable odors. Diuretics should only be used under medical supervision to avoid dehydration.

- **Absorbent Materials**: Using absorbent dressings or undergarments can help capture and contain odors emanating from sweat, reducing their spread.

Clinical Considerations

Healthcare providers should address odor-related concerns to ensure patient compliance and comfort:

- **Patient Counseling**: Discuss the inevitability of odor with patients and provide practical strategies for managing it. This includes tips on hygiene, use of absorbent materials, and timing of applications.

- **Formulation Adjustments**: Customize DMSO formulations to include odor-masking components based on patient preferences and sensitivities.

- **Supportive Measures**: Offer additional supportive measures, such as recommending specific laundry detergents or air fresheners that can help neutralize odors in the patient's environment.

Combined Management of Skin Irritation and Odor

In many cases, skin irritation and odor may coexist, particularly with higher concentrations of DMSO. An integrated approach to managing these side effects can enhance overall patient experience and adherence to therapy:

- **Balanced Formulations**: Develop formulations that optimize the therapeutic concentration of DMSO while incorporating agents that mitigate both skin irritation and odor.

- **Sequential Application**: Apply buffering agents or emollients immediately after DMSO to soothe the skin and create a barrier that may reduce local DMS metabolism and subsequent odor.

- **Comprehensive Monitoring**: Implement a holistic monitoring strategy that assesses both dermatological health and odor management, allowing for timely interventions and adjustments to the treatment regimen.

Managing the Garlic-like Smell

Introduction

One of the most distinctive and frequently reported side effects of Dimethyl sulfoxide (DMSO) use is its characteristic garlic-like odor. This odor, primarily resulting from the metabolic conversion of DMSO to dimethyl sulfide (DMS) and other sulfur-containing compounds, can pose challenges in both clinical and personal settings. Effective management of this odor is essential to enhance patient compliance, improve quality of life, and ensure the continued therapeutic use of DMSO. This section explores scientifically grounded strategies for mitigating the garlic-like smell associated with DMSO, examining both preventive and responsive measures, and highlighting best practices supported by research.

Understanding the Source of the Odor

Metabolic Conversion

- **Biochemical Pathways**: Upon administration, DMSO is metabolized in the liver through oxidative pathways, leading to the formation of dimethyl sulfide (DMS) and other volatile sulfur compounds. These metabolites are excreted via the respiratory system (breath) and urinary tract, resulting in the distinctive garlic-like odor.

- **Systemic and Local Metabolism**: Both systemic metabolism and local conversion at the site of application contribute to odor production. For topical applications, skin microbiota can further metabolize DMSO, enhancing the emission of sulfur compounds.

Preventive Strategies

Dose Optimization

- **Lower Concentrations**: Utilizing the lowest effective concentration of DMSO can reduce the extent of its metabolic conversion to odor-causing compounds. Studies indicate that lower concentrations (10-30%) are associated with milder odors compared to higher concentrations (50-70%).

- **Gradual Titration**: Introducing DMSO gradually allows the body to adjust its metabolic processes, potentially minimizing sudden spikes in DMS production and associated odors.

Timing of Application

- **Scheduled Applications**: Applying DMSO during times when odor is less socially disruptive, such as evenings or overnight, can help manage the perception of the garlic-like smell. This approach reduces the likelihood of odor interfering with daily social interactions.

- **Extended Wear Periods**: Allowing DMSO formulations to dry completely before covering the treated area can limit the volatilization of sulfur compounds, thereby reducing odor intensity.

Formulation Adjustments

- **Odor-Neutralizing Agents**: Incorporating odor-neutralizing agents or fragrances into DMSO formulations can mask or diminish the garlic-like smell. Ingredients such as essential oils (e.g., lavender, eucalyptus) or commercially available odor-neutralizing compounds can be effective.

- **Buffered Formulations**: Adjusting the pH of DMSO solutions to a range that minimizes DMS metabolism can reduce the formation of odor-causing compounds. Typically, maintaining a slightly acidic to neutral pH (5.5-7.0) is optimal.

Enhanced Ventilation

- **Airflow Management**: Ensuring adequate ventilation in areas where DMSO is applied can help disperse volatile sulfur compounds, thereby reducing the concentration of odor in the immediate environment.

- **Use of Air Purifiers**: Employing air purifiers equipped with activated carbon filters can effectively capture and neutralize sulfur compounds, mitigating the persistence of the garlic-like odor.

Responsive Measures

Personal Hygiene Practices

- **Regular Washing**: Encouraging thorough washing of treated areas can remove residual DMSO and its metabolites, thereby reducing odor. Using mild, fragrance-free cleansers can prevent further irritation while effectively managing odor.

- **Oral Hygiene**: Since DMSO metabolites are excreted via the breath, maintaining good oral hygiene through regular brushing, flossing, and the use of mouthwashes can help minimize the garlic-like odor emanating from the mouth.

Dietary Modifications

- **Sulfur-Reducing Foods**: Incorporating foods that reduce sulfur compound production in the body, such as citrus fruits, leafy greens, and probiotics, can help mitigate the intensity of DMSO-induced odors.

- **Hydration**: Adequate fluid intake supports the efficient excretion of DMSO metabolites, thereby reducing their concentration and associated odors.

Use of Absorbent Materials

- **Odor-Absorbing Dressings**: Applying absorbent dressings or barrier films over DMSO-treated areas can capture and contain volatilized sulfur compounds, limiting their spread and reducing perceptible odor.

- **Garment Selection**: Wearing breathable, moisture-wicking fabrics can help absorb sweat and reduce the concentration of odor-causing compounds on the skin.

Pharmacological Interventions

- **Antioxidants**: Administering antioxidants alongside DMSO may help reduce oxidative stress and limit the formation of volatile sulfur compounds, thereby decreasing odor intensity.

- **Chelating Agents**: In specific cases, chelating agents that bind sulfur compounds could be explored to reduce the bioavailability of odor-causing metabolites. However, this approach requires thorough investigation to ensure safety and efficacy.

Clinical Considerations

Patient Education and Counseling

- **Informing Patients**: Educating patients about the inevitability of DMSO-induced odor and the strategies available to manage it can improve compliance and reduce anxiety related to odor concerns.

- **Behavioral Strategies**: Advising patients on behavioral modifications, such as avoiding tight clothing or environments with poor ventilation, can help minimize odor perception.

Monitoring and Follow-Up

- **Regular Assessments**: Conducting periodic evaluations to monitor the severity of odor and the effectiveness of mitigation strategies allows for timely adjustments to treatment protocols.

- **Feedback Mechanisms**: Establishing channels for patient feedback regarding odor issues can inform personalized management plans and enhance overall treatment satisfaction.

Alternative Formulations

- **Encapsulated DMSO**: Exploring encapsulation technologies that release DMSO in a controlled manner may reduce the immediate volatilization of sulfur compounds, thereby mitigating odor.

- **Combination Therapies**: Utilizing DMSO in combination with other therapeutic agents that either mask or neutralize odors can offer a balanced approach to managing side effects while maintaining therapeutic efficacy.

Herxheimer Reaction and Healing Crisis

Introduction

When initiating therapies aimed at eliminating pathogens or facilitating significant physiological changes, patients may experience transient exacerbations of symptoms known as the Herxheimer Reaction and Healing Crisis. These phenomena, while often misunderstood, play critical roles in the overall healing process. Understanding their manifestations, underlying mechanisms, and management strategies is essential for practitioners utilizing Dimethyl sulfoxide (DMSO) in therapeutic protocols. This section elucidates the nature of the Herxheimer Reaction and Healing Crisis within the context of DMSO usage, providing a comprehensive guide to recognizing, differentiating, and managing these responses to optimize patient outcomes.

Understanding Herxheimer Reaction

Definition

The Herxheimer Reaction, commonly referred to as a "Herx reaction," is an acute, transient inflammatory response that occurs shortly after the initiation of antimicrobial or detoxifying therapies. It is characterized by a temporary worsening of symptoms due to the rapid die-off of pathogens, leading to the release of endotoxins and other inflammatory mediators.

Mechanisms

- **Pathogen Lysis**: The sudden destruction of a large number of pathogens releases intracellular components, including endotoxins, into the host's system.

- **Immune Activation**: These released components act as pathogen-associated molecular patterns (PAMPs), triggering the host's immune system to mount an inflammatory response.

- **Cytokine Release**: Elevated levels of pro-inflammatory cytokines such as interleukin-6 (IL-6) and tumor necrosis factor-alpha (TNF-α) contribute to systemic inflammatory symptoms.

Symptoms

- **Systemic**: Fever, chills, headache, muscle aches, and fatigue.

- **Local**: Increased redness, swelling, and pain at the site of pathogen elimination or therapy application.

- **Gastrointestinal**: Nausea, vomiting, and diarrhea may occur in severe cases.

Triggers

- **Antimicrobial Therapies**: Initiation of antibiotics, antifungals, or antiparasitic agents.

- **Detoxifying Agents**: Use of substances like DMSO that facilitate the removal of toxins or dead pathogens from tissues.

Understanding Healing Crisis

Definition

A Healing Crisis, often termed a "healing reaction," refers to a temporary intensification of symptoms experienced by individuals undergoing therapies that induce significant physiological changes. Unlike the Herxheimer Reaction, which is primarily associated with pathogen die-off, a Healing Crisis encompasses a broader spectrum of symptom exacerbations related to the body's natural detoxification and healing processes.

Mechanisms

- **Detoxification Processes**: Enhanced elimination of toxins from tissues and organs can lead to transient symptoms as the body adjusts to improved metabolic functions.
- **Immune System Modulation**: Therapies that stimulate the immune system may result in temporary increases in inflammatory markers as the body combats residual pathogens or toxins.
- **Cellular Regeneration**: Increased cellular turnover and repair activities can manifest as heightened sensations of discomfort or fatigue.

Symptoms

- **Systemic**: Fatigue, malaise, headaches, and muscle soreness.
- **Psychological**: Mood swings, irritability, and temporary cognitive disturbances.
- **Gastrointestinal**: Increased bowel movements, bloating, or changes in appetite.

Triggers

- **Holistic Therapies**: Practices such as acupuncture, herbal medicine, and nutrient supplementation.
- **Detoxification Protocols**: Use of DMSO in regimens aimed at enhancing detoxification and cellular repair.

Herxheimer Reaction in the Context of DMSO

Mechanisms Specific to DMSO

DMSO's role as a solvent and carrier agent can potentiate the Herxheimer Reaction by enhancing the penetration and efficacy of antimicrobial agents or facilitating the removal of dead pathogens from tissues. This increased efficacy can lead to a more pronounced die-off of pathogens, thereby intensifying the Herxheimer Reaction.

Clinical Scenarios

- **Infections**: When DMSO is used adjunctively with antibiotics to treat chronic infections such as Lyme disease or interstitial cystitis, the rapid elimination of pathogens may precipitate a Herxheimer Reaction.
- **Inflammatory Conditions**: In autoimmune or inflammatory disorders, DMSO's anti-inflammatory properties may alter immune responses, potentially triggering transient inflammatory exacerbations.

Healing Crisis in the Context of DMSO

Mechanisms Specific to DMSO

DMSO's capacity to enhance cellular permeability and facilitate detoxification processes can contribute to a Healing Crisis by promoting the rapid elimination of cellular debris, toxins, and inflammatory mediators. This accelerated detoxification can overwhelm the body's adaptive mechanisms, resulting in temporary symptom intensification.

Clinical Scenarios

- **Detoxification Protocols**: In protocols where DMSO is employed to expedite the removal of heavy metals or other toxins, the sudden influx of detoxified substances into the bloodstream may trigger a Healing Crisis.

- **Regenerative Therapies**: When used in regenerative treatments, such as promoting tissue repair in musculoskeletal injuries, DMSO may enhance cellular activity to a degree that temporarily amplifies discomfort or fatigue.

Differentiating Herxheimer Reaction and Healing Crisis

Herxheimer Reaction

- **Primary Cause**: Pathogen die-off and release of endotoxins.
- **Symptom Onset**: Typically occurs shortly after initiating antimicrobial therapy.
- **Focus**: Acute inflammatory response due to rapid pathogen elimination.

Healing Crisis

- **Primary Cause**: Enhanced detoxification and physiological adjustments.
- **Symptom Onset**: Can occur at various stages of therapy, not limited to pathogen elimination.
- **Focus**: Broader physiological adaptations involving detoxification and cellular repair.

Management Strategies

Immediate Steps

- **Assessment**: Differentiate between Herxheimer Reaction and Healing Crisis based on symptom onset, associated therapies, and clinical presentation.
- **Symptom Monitoring**: Continuously monitor vital signs and symptom severity to determine the appropriate intervention level.

Supportive Care

- **Hydration**: Encourage increased fluid intake to facilitate the excretion of toxins and metabolites.
- **Rest and Nutrition**: Ensure adequate rest and provide nutrient-dense foods to support the body's healing processes.
- **Anti-inflammatory Agents**: Use non-steroidal anti-inflammatory drugs (NSAIDs) or natural anti-inflammatory supplements to alleviate acute inflammation, if appropriate and under medical supervision.

Adjusting DMSO Therapy

- **Dose Reduction**: Temporarily lowering the dose of DMSO may help mitigate severe reactions while maintaining therapeutic benefits.
- **Frequency Modification**: Adjusting the frequency of DMSO administration can provide the body with adequate time to adapt to physiological changes.
- **Therapeutic Pauses**: Implementing short breaks in therapy can allow the body to stabilize and recover from transient symptom exacerbations.

Patient Education

- **Expectation Management**: Inform patients about the possibility of experiencing Herxheimer Reactions or Healing Crises and the typical duration and severity of these responses.
- **Self-Monitoring Techniques**: Teach patients to recognize early signs of adverse reactions and the importance of reporting significant symptom changes promptly.
- **Coping Strategies**: Provide strategies for managing discomfort, such as relaxation techniques, gentle exercise, and supportive therapies like massage or acupuncture.

Clinical Considerations

When to Seek Medical Attention

- **Severe Symptoms**: Immediate medical intervention is necessary if symptoms include high fever, severe pain, significant swelling, or signs of allergic reactions.

- **Prolonged Reactions**: Persistent or worsening symptoms beyond the expected duration warrant further evaluation to rule out complications or alternative diagnoses.

Patient-Specific Factors

- **Underlying Health Conditions**: Consider pre-existing health conditions that may predispose patients to more severe reactions, such as autoimmune disorders, chronic infections, or compromised organ function.

- **Medication Interactions**: Evaluate potential interactions between DMSO and other medications the patient is taking, as these can influence the severity and management of reactions.

Contraindications and When Not to Use DMSO

Introduction

While Dimethyl sulfoxide (DMSO) is recognized for its versatile therapeutic applications, it is not universally suitable for all individuals or conditions. Understanding the contraindications and scenarios where DMSO should be avoided is crucial to ensure patient safety and optimize therapeutic outcomes. This section delineates the specific medical conditions, patient populations, and circumstances under which the use of DMSO is contraindicated, providing a comprehensive overview grounded in scientific evidence.

Absolute Contraindications

Absolute contraindications are conditions or factors that pose a significant risk of severe adverse effects if DMSO is administered. In such cases, the use of DMSO is strictly prohibited.

Pregnancy and Lactation

- **Rationale**: There is limited data on the safety of DMSO during pregnancy and breastfeeding. Animal studies have indicated potential teratogenic effects at high doses, and the transdermal absorption of DMSO can facilitate the transfer of other compounds into fetal circulation or breast milk.

- **Implications**: DMSO should be avoided in pregnant and lactating individuals to prevent potential harm to the fetus or infant.

Hypersensitivity and Allergic Reactions

- **Rationale**: Individuals with a known hypersensitivity or allergic reaction to DMSO or any of its derivatives are at risk of severe allergic responses, including anaphylaxis.

- **Implications**: A history of allergic reactions to DMSO mandates the avoidance of its use to prevent life-threatening allergic events.

Severe Liver or Kidney Dysfunction

- **Rationale**: DMSO is metabolized primarily in the liver and excreted via the kidneys. Severe impairment of these organs can lead to accumulation of DMSO and its metabolites, increasing the risk of toxicity and adverse effects.

- **Implications**: Patients with significant hepatic or renal impairment should not be administered DMSO unless under strict medical supervision with careful dose adjustments.

Relative Contraindications

Relative contraindications are conditions where DMSO can be used with caution, typically requiring close monitoring or dose adjustments to mitigate potential risks.

Cardiovascular Disorders

- **Rationale**: DMSO can cause peripheral vasodilation and hypotension, which may exacerbate existing cardiovascular conditions such as heart failure, arrhythmias, or hypertension.

- **Implications**: In patients with cardiovascular disorders, DMSO should be used cautiously, with continuous monitoring of blood pressure and cardiac function.

Diabetes Mellitus

- **Rationale**: DMSO may affect blood glucose levels and insulin sensitivity, potentially complicating glycemic control in diabetic patients.

- **Implications**: Diabetic individuals receiving DMSO therapy should have their blood glucose levels closely monitored, and adjustments to diabetic medications may be necessary.

Seizure Disorders

- **Rationale**: DMSO has central nervous system (CNS) effects that could lower the seizure threshold, increasing the risk of seizure activity in susceptible individuals.

- **Implications**: Patients with a history of seizures should be evaluated carefully before initiating DMSO therapy, and CNS symptoms should be monitored during treatment.

Peripheral Neuropathy

- **Rationale**: DMSO can exacerbate existing nerve damage or neuropathic conditions due to its neurotoxic potential at high concentrations.

- **Implications**: In patients with peripheral neuropathy, lower doses of DMSO should be considered, and neurological symptoms should be closely observed.

Specific Medical Conditions

Certain medical conditions inherently pose risks when treated with DMSO, necessitating its avoidance or the implementation of stringent safeguards.

Interstitial Cystitis

- **Rationale**: While DMSO is approved by the U.S. Food and Drug Administration (FDA) for intravesical use in interstitial cystitis, systemic use in individuals with this condition may lead to exacerbated symptoms or adverse reactions.

- **Implications**: Systemic DMSO therapy in interstitial cystitis patients should be approached with caution, adhering strictly to approved intravesical application protocols.

Active Infections

- **Rationale**: DMSO's immune-modulating effects can potentially interfere with the body's natural response to active infections, possibly hindering pathogen clearance.

- **Implications**: The presence of active bacterial, viral, or fungal infections is a relative contraindication, warranting careful consideration and possible alternative therapies.

Hemorrhagic Conditions

- **Rationale**: DMSO has antiplatelet effects that can impair blood clotting mechanisms, increasing the risk of bleeding in individuals with hemorrhagic disorders or those on anticoagulant therapy.

- **Implications**: In patients with bleeding disorders or those receiving anticoagulants, the use of DMSO should be avoided or closely monitored to prevent hemorrhagic complications.

Drug Interactions

DMSO can interact with various medications, altering their pharmacokinetics and pharmacodynamics, which may lead to unintended side effects or diminished therapeutic efficacy.

Anticoagulants and Antiplatelet Agents

- **Rationale**: DMSO's antiplatelet effects can potentiate the actions of anticoagulants and antiplatelet agents, increasing the risk of bleeding.

- **Implications**: Concurrent use of DMSO with these medications should be avoided or managed with careful dose adjustments and monitoring of coagulation parameters.

Immunosuppressants

- **Rationale**: DMSO has immunomodulatory properties that may interfere with the efficacy of immunosuppressive drugs, potentially leading to suboptimal management of autoimmune conditions or organ transplant recipients.
- **Implications**: Patients on immunosuppressants should consult their healthcare provider before starting DMSO therapy to evaluate potential interactions and adjust treatment plans accordingly.

Chemotherapeutic Agents

- **Rationale**: DMSO can alter the absorption and distribution of chemotherapeutic drugs, potentially impacting their efficacy and toxicity profiles.
- **Implications**: Coordination with oncologists is essential when combining DMSO with chemotherapy to ensure therapeutic effectiveness and minimize adverse interactions.

Situational Contraindications

Certain scenarios necessitate the avoidance of DMSO to prevent complications or ensure the integrity of treatment outcomes.

Recent Surgery or Trauma

- **Rationale**: DMSO's penetrative properties can interfere with wound healing or exacerbate inflammation in recently operated or traumatized tissues.
- **Implications**: Postoperative and post-traumatic patients should refrain from using DMSO on affected areas until adequate healing has occurred and medical clearance is obtained.

Use with Photodynamic Therapy

- **Rationale**: DMSO may increase the skin's sensitivity to light, heightening the risk of phototoxic reactions when combined with photodynamic therapy.
- **Implications**: Avoid simultaneous use of DMSO and photodynamic agents to prevent severe skin reactions and phototoxicity.

Pregnancy-Related Complications

- **Rationale**: Beyond general pregnancy contraindications, specific complications such as preeclampsia or gestational diabetes may interact adversely with DMSO's pharmacological effects.
- **Implications**: In cases of pregnancy-related complications, DMSO use should be contraindicated unless unequivocally deemed necessary by a healthcare provider with specialized expertise.

Chapter 8: DMSO and Integrative Medicine

Combining DMSO with Conventional Treatments

Introduction

Dimethyl sulfoxide (DMSO) has garnered attention in both alternative and complementary medicine due to its multifaceted therapeutic properties, including anti-inflammatory, analgesic, and solvent capabilities. In recent years, there has been a growing interest in integrating DMSO with conventional medical treatments to enhance therapeutic efficacy and patient outcomes. Combining DMSO with established medical interventions can potentially amplify the benefits of standard therapies, improve drug delivery, and offer synergistic effects in managing various health conditions. This section explores the scientific foundations, applications, evidence, safety considerations, and best practices associated with the integration of DMSO into conventional treatment regimens.

Synergistic Enhancement of Drug Delivery

Mechanisms of Enhanced Penetration

DMSO is renowned for its ability to disrupt cellular membranes and enhance the permeability of biological barriers. When combined with conventional topical medications, DMSO can facilitate deeper and more uniform penetration of active pharmaceutical ingredients (APIs) into target tissues. This mechanism is particularly advantageous in the administration of anti-inflammatory drugs, analgesics, and antibiotics applied to the skin or mucosal surfaces.

- **Transdermal Transport**: DMSO modifies the lipid structure of the stratum corneum, increasing skin permeability and allowing for more efficient transdermal drug delivery.

- **Carrier Solvent**: Acting as a carrier solvent, DMSO can dissolve hydrophilic and hydrophobic drugs, ensuring their uniform distribution and sustained release within the tissue.

Clinical Applications

- **Topical Steroids and Anti-Inflammatories**: Combining DMSO with corticosteroids or non-steroidal anti-inflammatory drugs (NSAIDs) can enhance their anti-inflammatory effects in conditions like psoriasis, eczema, and rheumatoid arthritis.

- **Antibiotic Therapies**: DMSO can improve the efficacy of topical antibiotics in treating skin infections by ensuring better drug distribution and retention at the site of infection.

Synergistic Anti-Inflammatory and Analgesic Effects

Dual Mechanistic Pathways

DMSO and conventional anti-inflammatory or analgesic medications often operate through distinct yet complementary biological pathways. This dual action can result in a more comprehensive reduction of inflammation and pain compared to either agent alone.

- **DMSO's Role**: DMSO inhibits the synthesis of pro-inflammatory cytokines and prostaglandins while scavenging free radicals, thereby reducing oxidative stress and inflammation.

- **Conventional Medications**: Drugs such as NSAIDs inhibit cyclooxygenase enzymes (COX-1 and COX-2), decreasing prostaglandin synthesis and thereby alleviating pain and inflammation.

Enhanced Therapeutic Outcomes

- **Reduced Dosage Requirements**: The synergistic effects may allow for lower doses of conventional medications, minimizing potential side effects while maintaining or enhancing therapeutic efficacy.

- **Improved Symptom Management**: Patients may experience more rapid and sustained relief from symptoms, improving overall quality of life and functional abilities.

Integration with Chemotherapeutic Agents

Improved Chemotherapy Delivery

DMSO's solvent properties can enhance the solubility and stability of chemotherapeutic agents, facilitating their effective delivery to cancerous tissues. This is particularly relevant in topical chemotherapy for skin cancers or intravesical therapy for bladder cancer.

- **Enhanced Solubility**: DMSO can dissolve poorly water-soluble chemotherapeutic drugs, ensuring their bioavailability and therapeutic action.

- **Targeted Delivery**: By increasing tissue permeability, DMSO aids in the targeted delivery of chemotherapeutic agents, potentially reducing systemic toxicity and improving local efficacy.

Clinical Evidence

- **Topical Chemotherapy**: Studies have demonstrated that DMSO-enhanced formulations of drugs like 5-fluorouracil exhibit improved penetration and efficacy in treating basal cell carcinoma and other skin malignancies.

- **Intravesical Therapy**: In bladder cancer treatment, DMSO used as a carrier for chemotherapeutic agents has shown promise in enhancing drug retention and therapeutic outcomes.

Potential Interactions and Safety Considerations

Pharmacokinetic and Pharmacodynamic Interactions

Combining DMSO with conventional medications can alter the pharmacokinetics (absorption, distribution, metabolism, excretion) and pharmacodynamics (drug effects and mechanisms) of the co-administered drugs. Understanding these interactions is crucial to prevent adverse effects and optimize therapeutic outcomes.

- **Increased Absorption**: DMSO's permeability-enhancing effects can lead to higher systemic absorption of co-administered drugs, potentially increasing their efficacy and toxicity.

- **Altered Metabolism**: DMSO may influence liver enzymes responsible for drug metabolism, affecting the breakdown and clearance of medications.

Adverse Effects and Mitigation

- **Skin Irritation**: While DMSO enhances drug delivery, it can also increase the risk of skin irritation from topical medications. Mitigation strategies include using lower concentrations of DMSO, incorporating emollients, and applying formulations sparingly.

- **Systemic Toxicity**: Enhanced systemic absorption of drugs can lead to unintended side effects. Close monitoring of drug levels and patient symptoms is essential, particularly when using potent medications.

Best Practices for Combining DMSO with Conventional Treatments

Comprehensive Patient Evaluation

Before integrating DMSO into a conventional treatment regimen, a thorough patient evaluation is necessary to assess suitability and identify potential risks.

- **Medical History**: Review the patient's medical history for conditions that may contraindicate DMSO use, such as liver or kidney dysfunction, hypersensitivity to DMSO, or concurrent use of medications that may interact adversely.

- **Medication Review**: Analyze current medications to identify potential interactions and adjust dosages accordingly.

Gradual Introduction and Titration

Introducing DMSO gradually allows for the assessment of patient tolerance and the minimization of adverse effects.

- **Starting Low**: Begin with lower concentrations of DMSO and conventional medications, gradually increasing as tolerated based on therapeutic response and absence of adverse reactions.

- **Monitoring**: Implement regular monitoring protocols to track patient progress, drug levels, and the emergence of any side effects.

Formulation Optimization

Developing optimized formulations that balance DMSO's penetration-enhancing properties with patient comfort and safety is critical.

- **Concentration Balance**: Use the minimum effective concentration of DMSO to achieve desired drug delivery without causing excessive irritation or systemic absorption.
- **Additives and Stabilizers**: Incorporate skin-soothing agents, antioxidants, or preservatives as necessary to enhance formulation stability and patient tolerability.

Patient Education and Compliance

Educating patients about the rationale for combining DMSO with conventional treatments and instructing them on proper application techniques can enhance compliance and treatment outcomes.

- **Instruction on Use**: Provide clear instructions on how to apply DMSO-containing formulations, emphasizing areas such as dosage, frequency, and application sites.
- **Awareness of Side Effects**: Inform patients about potential side effects, including skin irritation and odor, and educate them on strategies to manage these issues.

Collaboration with Healthcare Providers

Effective integration of DMSO into conventional treatment plans requires collaboration among healthcare providers to ensure coordinated and comprehensive patient care.

- **Interdisciplinary Approach**: Engage dermatologists, oncologists, rheumatologists, and other specialists as needed to tailor DMSO integration based on specific clinical scenarios.
- **Regular Communication**: Maintain open lines of communication to adjust treatment protocols based on patient responses and emerging clinical data.

Case Studies and Clinical Evidence

Case Study 1: Enhanced Topical Steroid Therapy in Psoriasis

A study involving patients with moderate to severe psoriasis demonstrated that combining DMSO with topical corticosteroids significantly improved lesion clearance rates and reduced treatment duration compared to corticosteroids alone. The enhanced penetration facilitated by DMSO allowed for lower steroid concentrations, minimizing potential side effects such as skin atrophy.

Case Study 2: Improved Outcomes in Osteoarthritis Management

In a clinical trial with patients suffering from osteoarthritis, the application of DMSO-enhanced NSAID gels resulted in greater pain relief and improved joint mobility compared to standard NSAID gels. The synergistic anti-inflammatory effects contributed to a more effective management of osteoarthritic symptoms.

Clinical Evidence in Oncology

Research on intravesical therapy for bladder cancer has shown that DMSO as a carrier solvent improves the retention and efficacy of chemotherapeutic agents like doxorubicin, leading to higher rates of tumor regression and lower recurrence rates.

DMSO in Alternative and Naturopathic Medicine

Introduction

Dimethyl sulfoxide (DMSO) has long been embraced within alternative and naturopathic medicine circles for its purported therapeutic benefits. Unlike conventional medical settings where DMSO is primarily utilized for its anti-inflammatory and analgesic properties, alternative and naturopathic practitioners leverage its multifaceted capabilities to address a broader spectrum of health concerns. This section explores the integration of DMSO within alternative and naturopathic frameworks, elucidates its synergistic use with other natural therapies, examines the underlying philosophies, reviews empirical evidence supporting its use, discusses safety considerations unique to this context, and highlights future directions for research and application.

Philosophical Foundations in Naturopathic Medicine

Holistic Healing Approach

Naturopathic medicine emphasizes a holistic approach, focusing on the interconnectedness of the body's systems and the promotion of overall wellness. DMSO fits within this paradigm due to its ability to act on multiple physiological pathways simultaneously. Practitioners view DMSO not merely as a symptomatic treatment but as a facilitator of systemic healing and detoxification.

Support for the Body's Natural Healing Processes

Naturopathic philosophy advocates for supporting and enhancing the body's intrinsic ability to heal itself. DMSO is employed to optimize cellular function and enhance the efficacy of other natural remedies, thereby amplifying the body's regenerative capabilities. Its role as a carrier solvent aligns with the naturopathic emphasis on maximizing the bioavailability of therapeutic agents.

Integration with Other Alternative Therapies

Herbal Medicine

DMSO is frequently combined with various herbal extracts to enhance their penetration and efficacy. For instance, when paired with anti-inflammatory herbs like turmeric (Curcuma longa) or boswellia (Boswellia serrata), DMSO can facilitate deeper tissue absorption, potentially amplifying their therapeutic effects in conditions such as arthritis and chronic pain.

Homeopathy

In homeopathic practices, DMSO is sometimes used as a solvent to prepare highly diluted remedies, leveraging its ability to enhance the bioavailability of homeopathic agents. This combination aims to improve the therapeutic outcomes of homeopathic treatments by ensuring that active compounds are more effectively delivered to target tissues.

Acupuncture

DMSO may be used adjunctively with acupuncture to augment the treatment's effectiveness. By applying DMSO to acupuncture points, practitioners believe that it can enhance the delivery of healing agents to specific meridians, potentially increasing the benefits of acupuncture sessions in pain management and systemic balance.

Nutritional Supplements

DMSO is often integrated with nutritional supplements such as vitamins and minerals to enhance their absorption and efficacy. For example, combining DMSO with Vitamin C can potentiate its antioxidant effects, supporting immune function and cellular protection.

Specific Conditions Addressed in Alternative Medicine

Chronic Inflammatory Diseases

Naturopathic practitioners utilize DMSO to manage chronic inflammatory conditions such as rheumatoid arthritis, inflammatory bowel disease, and chronic prostatitis. Its anti-inflammatory properties, combined with enhanced drug delivery, aim to reduce inflammation and alleviate associated symptoms more effectively than conventional therapies alone.

Detoxification Protocols

DMSO is a cornerstone in many detoxification regimens within naturopathic medicine. It is believed to aid in the elimination of toxins and heavy metals from the body by enhancing cellular permeability and facilitating the transport of detoxifying agents to tissues.

Skin Conditions

Beyond conventional uses, alternative practitioners employ DMSO in treating a variety of dermatological issues, including eczema, psoriasis, and acne. Its ability to deliver topical treatments more effectively is leveraged to improve skin health and expedite the healing of wounds and lesions.

Pain Management

Chronic pain syndromes, including fibromyalgia and neuropathic pain, are commonly addressed with DMSO in alternative medicine. Its analgesic properties, coupled with enhanced delivery of pain-relieving agents, provide a comprehensive approach to pain management.

Empirical Evidence Supporting Alternative Use

Preclinical Studies

Preclinical research has demonstrated DMSO's efficacy in enhancing the bioavailability of various therapeutic agents. Animal studies indicate that DMSO can improve the absorption and distribution of herbal extracts, leading to more pronounced therapeutic outcomes in models of inflammation and pain.

Clinical Studies

While robust clinical trials within conventional medicine are limited, some studies in alternative medicine settings suggest potential benefits of DMSO integration. For example, clinical observations in patients with interstitial cystitis have shown improved symptom relief when DMSO is used alongside other naturopathic treatments. However, more rigorous, peer-reviewed studies are necessary to substantiate these findings.

Case Reports and Anecdotal Evidence

Numerous case reports and anecdotal accounts from naturopathic practitioners highlight successful outcomes using DMSO in combination with other alternative therapies. These narratives often emphasize improved symptom management and enhanced quality of life, though they lack the methodological rigor of controlled studies.

Safety Considerations in Alternative Use

Concentration and Dosage

In alternative and naturopathic settings, DMSO is typically used at concentrations ranging from 10% to 50%, depending on the condition being treated and the modality of administration. It is imperative to adhere to recommended dosages to minimize the risk of adverse effects such as skin irritation and systemic toxicity.

Potential for Enhanced Side Effects

The synergistic use of DMSO with other natural agents can potentiate both therapeutic effects and side effects. For instance, combining DMSO with potent anti-inflammatory herbs may increase the risk of gastrointestinal disturbances or liver strain. Practitioners must carefully evaluate the cumulative effects of combined therapies.

Individual Sensitivities and Allergies

Patients may exhibit individual sensitivities or allergic reactions to DMSO or concomitant natural therapies. Patch testing and gradual introduction of DMSO-containing formulations can help identify and mitigate allergic responses.

Regulatory and Quality Assurance

Ensuring the use of pharmaceutical-grade DMSO is crucial to avoid contamination and impurities that could exacerbate side effects. Alternative practitioners should source DMSO from reputable suppliers and adhere to quality assurance standards to maintain formulation integrity.

The Role of Diet and Lifestyle

Introduction

The efficacy of Dimethyl sulfoxide (DMSO) as a therapeutic agent can be significantly influenced by an individual's diet and lifestyle. While DMSO possesses intrinsic pharmacological properties that contribute to its therapeutic effects, optimizing these effects through dietary and lifestyle modifications can enhance overall outcomes, mitigate potential side effects, and support the body's natural healing processes. This section explores the interplay between diet, lifestyle factors, and DMSO therapy, providing evidence-based recommendations to maximize the benefits of DMSO treatment.

Dietary Considerations

Nutrient-Rich Diet

A balanced, nutrient-dense diet supports the body's ability to respond effectively to DMSO therapy. Adequate intake of essential vitamins and minerals is crucial for maintaining cellular health and facilitating the body's detoxification pathways.

- **Antioxidants**: Consuming foods high in antioxidants, such as berries, leafy greens, nuts, and seeds, can complement DMSO's antioxidant properties by neutralizing free radicals and reducing oxidative stress.

- **Hydration**: Adequate fluid intake is essential when using DMSO, as it facilitates the excretion of metabolites and supports overall cellular function. Aim for at least 8-10 glasses of water daily, incorporating herbal teas and electrolyte-rich beverages as needed.

- **Protein Intake**: Sufficient protein supports tissue repair and regeneration, which can be beneficial in conjunction with DMSO's role in enhancing drug delivery to tissues.

Detoxification-Supportive Foods

Incorporating foods that aid the body's natural detoxification processes can enhance the efficacy of DMSO therapy by promoting the elimination of toxins and supporting liver function.

- **Cruciferous Vegetables**: Vegetables like broccoli, cauliflower, and Brussels sprouts contain compounds that support liver detoxification enzymes, enhancing the body's ability to process and eliminate DMSO metabolites.

- **Fiber-Rich Foods**: High-fiber foods such as whole grains, legumes, and vegetables promote gastrointestinal health and facilitate the removal of toxins through the digestive system.

- **Herbs and Spices**: Incorporating herbs like cilantro and spices such as turmeric can support detoxification and reduce inflammation, synergizing with DMSO's anti-inflammatory effects.

Avoiding Pro-Inflammatory Foods

Minimizing the intake of pro-inflammatory foods can reduce the overall inflammatory burden on the body, allowing DMSO's anti-inflammatory properties to function more effectively.

- **Processed Foods**: Reduce consumption of processed and high-sugar foods that can exacerbate inflammation and oxidative stress.

- **Saturated and Trans Fats**: Limit intake of saturated and trans fats found in fried foods, certain dairy products, and baked goods, as they can contribute to systemic inflammation.

- **Alcohol and Caffeine**: Excessive alcohol and caffeine intake can impair liver function and exacerbate dehydration, counteracting the benefits of DMSO therapy.

Lifestyle Factors

Physical Activity

Regular physical activity supports overall health and can enhance the therapeutic effects of DMSO by improving circulation, reducing inflammation, and promoting lymphatic drainage.

- **Aerobic Exercise**: Engaging in moderate aerobic activities such as walking, cycling, or swimming can enhance cardiovascular health and support the distribution of DMSO throughout the body.

- **Strength Training**: Incorporating strength training exercises helps maintain muscle mass and joint health, complementing DMSO's role in managing musculoskeletal conditions.

- **Flexibility and Mobility**: Practices such as yoga and stretching improve flexibility and reduce muscle tension, enhancing the overall effectiveness of DMSO in pain management.

Stress Management

Chronic stress can impair immune function and exacerbate inflammatory conditions, potentially diminishing the benefits of DMSO therapy. Effective stress management strategies are essential to support overall treatment outcomes.

- **Mindfulness and Meditation**: Incorporating mindfulness practices and meditation can reduce stress levels, lower cortisol production, and enhance mental well-being.

- **Adequate Sleep**: Ensuring 7-9 hours of quality sleep per night supports cellular repair, immune function, and overall health, optimizing the body's response to DMSO therapy.

- **Relaxation Techniques**: Engaging in relaxation techniques such as deep breathing exercises, progressive muscle relaxation, or tai chi can mitigate the physiological effects of stress.

Avoiding Toxins

Reducing exposure to environmental toxins can enhance the body's ability to detoxify and improve the efficacy of DMSO therapy.

- **Air Quality**: Maintain good indoor air quality by using air purifiers, avoiding smoking, and minimizing exposure to pollutants.

- **Chemical Exposure**: Limit the use of household chemicals and personal care products containing harmful substances that can burden the body's detoxification systems.

- **Safe Food Practices**: Choose organic produce when possible to reduce intake of pesticides and other contaminants, supporting overall health and detoxification processes.

Synergistic Supplements

Certain dietary supplements can work synergistically with DMSO to enhance its therapeutic effects and support overall health.

- **Vitamin C**: As a potent antioxidant, Vitamin C can complement DMSO's free radical scavenging abilities, supporting immune function and reducing oxidative stress.

- **Omega-3 Fatty Acids**: Found in fish oil and flaxseed oil, omega-3 fatty acids possess anti-inflammatory properties that can enhance the anti-inflammatory effects of DMSO.

- **B Vitamins**: B vitamins support energy metabolism and nervous system health, aiding in the body's overall response to DMSO therapy.

Anti-inflammatory Diets

Introduction

Anti-inflammatory diets are structured eating patterns designed to reduce chronic inflammation, a key underlying factor in numerous health conditions such as cardiovascular disease, diabetes, arthritis, and certain neurodegenerative disorders. Integrating an anti-inflammatory diet with Dimethyl sulfoxide (DMSO) therapy can potentially enhance therapeutic outcomes by synergistically targeting inflammatory pathways. This section delineates the principles of anti-inflammatory diets, explores specific dietary components that modulate inflammation, examines the interplay between these diets and DMSO therapy, reviews supporting scientific evidence, and provides practical guidelines for implementation.

Principles of Anti-inflammatory Diets

Dietary Patterns

Several well-established dietary patterns exhibit anti-inflammatory properties. These include:

- **Mediterranean Diet**: Emphasizes fruits, vegetables, whole grains, nuts, seeds, olive oil, and lean proteins such as fish. It limits red meat, processed foods, and refined sugars.

- **DASH Diet (Dietary Approaches to Stop Hypertension)**: Focuses on reducing sodium intake and increasing consumption of fruits, vegetables, whole grains, and low-fat dairy, while limiting saturated fats and sugars.

- **Plant-based Diets**: Prioritize plant-derived foods, including vegetables, fruits, legumes, nuts, and seeds, while minimizing or excluding animal products.

Macronutrient Composition

Anti-inflammatory diets typically feature:

- **Healthy Fats**: Rich in monounsaturated and polyunsaturated fats, particularly omega-3 fatty acids, which play a crucial role in modulating inflammatory responses.

- **Complex Carbohydrates**: High intake of fiber from whole grains, legumes, and vegetables supports gut health and reduces inflammatory markers.

- **Lean Proteins**: Preference for plant-based proteins and lean animal sources to minimize pro-inflammatory effects associated with high-fat animal products.

Micronutrient Density

These diets are abundant in vitamins, minerals, and phytochemicals that possess anti-inflammatory and antioxidant properties, contributing to the attenuation of oxidative stress and inflammatory signaling pathways.

Key Dietary Components and Their Anti-inflammatory Effects

Omega-3 Fatty Acids

- **Sources**: Fatty fish (salmon, mackerel, sardines), flaxseeds, chia seeds, walnuts, and algae-based supplements.

- **Mechanism**: Omega-3s inhibit the production of pro-inflammatory eicosanoids and cytokines while promoting the synthesis of anti-inflammatory resolvins and protectins.

- **Interaction with DMSO**: Enhanced cellular uptake facilitated by DMSO may increase the bioavailability of omega-3 fatty acids, amplifying their anti-inflammatory effects.

Antioxidant-Rich Foods

- **Sources**: Berries, dark leafy greens, nuts, seeds, and colorful vegetables.

- **Mechanism**: Antioxidants neutralize reactive oxygen species (ROS), reducing oxidative stress and subsequent inflammatory responses.

- **Interaction with DMSO**: DMSO's intrinsic antioxidant properties synergize with dietary antioxidants to provide a more comprehensive defense against oxidative damage.

Polyphenols and Flavonoids

- **Sources**: Green tea, dark chocolate, red wine (in moderation), berries, and citrus fruits.

- **Mechanism**: These compounds modulate inflammatory pathways by inhibiting nuclear factor-kappa B (NF-κB) and reducing the expression of pro-inflammatory genes.

- **Interaction with DMSO**: DMSO can enhance the cellular penetration of polyphenols, potentially increasing their efficacy in downregulating inflammatory signaling.

Fiber

- **Sources**: Whole grains, legumes, fruits, vegetables, and nuts.

- **Mechanism**: Dietary fiber promotes a healthy gut microbiome, which plays a pivotal role in regulating systemic inflammation through the production of short-chain fatty acids (SCFAs).

- **Interaction with DMSO**: Improved gut health through fiber intake can complement DMSO's systemic anti-inflammatory effects, fostering a balanced immune response.

Synergistic Interaction Between Anti-inflammatory Diets and DMSO Therapy

Enhanced Bioavailability of Anti-inflammatory Nutrients

DMSO's solvent properties facilitate the deeper penetration and enhanced absorption of bioactive nutrients from an anti-inflammatory diet. This increased bioavailability ensures that higher concentrations of anti-inflammatory agents reach target tissues, thereby potentiating their effects.

Complementary Mechanisms of Action

While DMSO directly inhibits pro-inflammatory cytokines and enhances drug delivery, anti-inflammatory diets provide a continuous supply of natural compounds that further suppress inflammatory pathways. This multi-faceted approach addresses inflammation from both pharmacological and nutritional angles, leading to more effective management of chronic inflammatory conditions.

Support for Cellular and Molecular Repair Processes

Anti-inflammatory diets supply essential nutrients that support cellular repair and regeneration. When combined with DMSO's ability to enhance cellular uptake, these nutrients can more effectively contribute to the restoration of tissue integrity and function.

Scientific Evidence Supporting the Combination

Preclinical Studies

Animal models have demonstrated that the combination of DMSO with omega-3 fatty acid supplementation results in a more pronounced reduction in inflammatory markers compared to either intervention alone. These studies highlight the potential for synergistic effects in modulating inflammation at the molecular level.

Clinical Research

Limited clinical studies suggest that patients undergoing DMSO therapy who adhere to an anti-inflammatory diet experience enhanced symptom relief and improved overall health outcomes. For instance, individuals with rheumatoid arthritis reported decreased joint pain and swelling when combining DMSO treatment with a Mediterranean diet, compared to those following the diet alone.

Mechanistic Insights

Research indicates that DMSO can upregulate the expression of genes involved in anti-inflammatory responses while downregulating pro-inflammatory genes. When paired with dietary polyphenols and omega-3s, this gene modulation is further amplified, leading to a more robust anti-inflammatory effect.

Practical Guidelines for Integrating Anti-inflammatory Diets with DMSO Therapy

Dietary Assessment and Planning

- **Individualized Nutrition Plans**: Develop tailored dietary plans that incorporate anti-inflammatory foods based on the patient's specific health conditions, preferences, and nutritional needs.

- **Nutrient Timing**: Coordinate meal timings with DMSO application schedules to maximize nutrient absorption and therapeutic synergy.

Implementation Strategies

- **Gradual Dietary Changes**: Introduce anti-inflammatory foods gradually to allow the body to adjust and to monitor for any adverse reactions or intolerances.

- **Meal Preparation**: Encourage the preparation of balanced meals that emphasize anti-inflammatory ingredients, ensuring consistency and adherence to the dietary plan.

- **Supplementation**: Where necessary, incorporate supplements such as omega-3 fatty acids, vitamin D, and antioxidants to ensure adequate intake of key anti-inflammatory nutrients.

Monitoring and Adjustment

- **Regular Monitoring**: Track inflammatory markers, symptom severity, and overall health status to assess the efficacy of the combined intervention.

- **Feedback Mechanisms**: Solicit patient feedback to identify challenges in adhering to the dietary plan and to make necessary adjustments for improved compliance and outcomes.

Education and Support

- **Nutritional Education**: Provide patients with information on the benefits of anti-inflammatory diets and practical tips for incorporating them into daily life.

- **Support Systems**: Facilitate access to dietitians, nutritionists, or support groups to assist patients in maintaining their dietary changes alongside DMSO therapy.

Raw Veganism and DMSO

Introduction

Raw Veganism is a dietary regimen that excludes all animal products and emphasizes the consumption of uncooked, unprocessed plant-based foods. Proponents of Raw Veganism argue that this diet maximizes nutrient intake, preserves enzymatic activity, and promotes optimal health by minimizing exposure to processed foods and potential toxins. When combined with Dimethyl sulfoxide (DMSO) therapy, Raw Veganism may offer complementary benefits by enhancing the body's natural detoxification processes and supporting cellular health. This section explores the principles of Raw Veganism, examines the potential synergistic interactions with DMSO, reviews relevant scientific evidence, discusses safety considerations, and provides practical guidelines for integrating these approaches to optimize therapeutic outcomes.

Principles of Raw Veganism

Dietary Framework

Raw Veganism is characterized by the following dietary principles:

- **Consumption of Uncooked Foods**: Foods are not heated above approximately 115°F (46°C) to preserve natural enzymes and nutrients.

- **Exclusion of Animal Products**: The diet eliminates all forms of meat, dairy, eggs, and other animal-derived ingredients.

- **Emphasis on Whole Foods**: Focus is on whole, minimally processed plant-based foods including fruits, vegetables, nuts, seeds, sprouted grains, and legumes.

- **Avoidance of Refined Sugars and Oils**: The diet steers clear of refined sugars, hydrogenated oils, and other processed additives.

Nutritional Focus

Raw Veganism prioritizes the intake of:

- **Vitamins and Minerals**: High in vitamins A, C, E, and K, as well as essential minerals like magnesium, potassium, and calcium.

- **Antioxidants and Phytochemicals**: Rich in compounds that combat oxidative stress and modulate inflammatory pathways.

- **Dietary Fiber**: Abundant in fruits, vegetables, and legumes, supporting gut health and promoting regular bowel movements.

- **Healthy Fats**: Derived from sources like avocados, nuts, seeds, and cold-pressed oils, providing essential fatty acids without the pro-inflammatory effects of saturated fats.

Synergistic Interaction Between Raw Veganism and DMSO Therapy

Enhanced Detoxification

Raw Veganism supports the body's natural detoxification mechanisms through:

- **High Antioxidant Intake**: Antioxidants from fruits and vegetables neutralize free radicals, reducing oxidative stress and complementing DMSO's own antioxidant properties.

- **Increased Fiber Consumption**: Dietary fiber promotes the elimination of toxins through the digestive system, enhancing the detoxifying effects of DMSO.

- **Hydration Support**: High water content in raw foods aids in maintaining optimal hydration levels, facilitating the excretion of DMSO metabolites.

Cellular Health and Repair

- **Enzymatic Preservation**: The consumption of uncooked foods preserves natural enzymes that aid in digestion and cellular repair, potentially enhancing the therapeutic effects of DMSO.

- **Nutrient Density**: The nutrient-rich profile of a Raw Vegan diet provides essential vitamins and minerals that support cellular integrity and function, synergizing with DMSO's role in cellular permeability and drug delivery.

Anti-inflammatory Effects

- **Phytochemical Synergy**: Phytochemicals in raw plant foods, such as polyphenols and flavonoids, work alongside DMSO's anti-inflammatory actions to more effectively reduce chronic inflammation.

- **Balanced Omega Fatty Acids**: The balance of omega-3 and omega-6 fatty acids in a Raw Vegan diet supports anti-inflammatory processes, complementing DMSO's modulation of cytokine production.

Scientific Evidence Supporting Raw Veganism and DMSO Integration

Preclinical Studies

- **Animal Models**: Studies in rodents have shown that diets high in raw plant-based foods can enhance the efficacy of anti-inflammatory agents, including solvents like DMSO, by improving overall metabolic health and reducing systemic inflammation.

- **Cellular Studies**: In vitro research indicates that the combination of plant-derived antioxidants and DMSO can synergistically protect cells from oxidative damage, promoting cellular longevity and function.

Clinical Research

- **Inflammatory Conditions**: Preliminary clinical observations suggest that patients with chronic inflammatory conditions, such as rheumatoid arthritis, experience improved symptom management when combining Raw Vegan diets with DMSO therapy. Enhanced nutrient intake and anti-inflammatory compounds from the diet complement DMSO's pharmacological effects.

- **Detoxification Protocols**: Clinical protocols that integrate Raw Veganism with DMSO detoxification regimens report more efficient toxin elimination and improved patient well-being, likely due to the combined effects of dietary fiber and DMSO's solvent properties.

Mechanistic Insights

- **Oxidative Stress Reduction**: Both Raw Veganism and DMSO independently reduce oxidative stress through distinct mechanisms—dietary antioxidants scavenge free radicals, while DMSO neutralizes reactive oxygen species. Their combined use provides a more comprehensive defense against oxidative damage.

- **Enhanced Nutrient Uptake**: DMSO's ability to increase cellular permeability can enhance the uptake of vitamins, minerals, and phytochemicals from a Raw Vegan diet, maximizing their therapeutic potential.

Practical Guidelines for Integrating Raw Veganism with DMSO Therapy

Dietary Assessment and Planning

- **Individualized Nutrition Plans**: Develop tailored Raw Vegan meal plans that ensure adequate intake of all essential nutrients, taking into account the patient's specific health conditions and therapeutic goals.

- **Supplementation**: Consider supplementing with nutrients that may be less abundant in a Raw Vegan diet, such as Vitamin B12, Vitamin D, and omega-3 fatty acids, to support overall health and complement DMSO therapy.

Implementation Strategies

- **Gradual Dietary Transition**: Introduce Raw Vegan foods gradually to allow the body to adapt, minimizing gastrointestinal discomfort and ensuring sustained adherence.

- **Meal Preparation Education**: Provide education on preparing balanced Raw Vegan meals, emphasizing variety and nutrient density to support therapeutic outcomes.

- **Hydration Focus**: Encourage the consumption of high-water-content raw foods and adequate fluid intake to support detoxification and facilitate the excretion of DMSO metabolites.

Monitoring and Adjustment

- **Regular Health Assessments**: Conduct periodic evaluations of nutritional status, inflammatory markers, and overall health to assess the efficacy of the combined intervention.

- **Symptom Tracking**: Implement symptom tracking to identify improvements or any adverse reactions, allowing for timely adjustments to the diet or DMSO dosage.

- **Feedback Mechanisms**: Establish channels for patient feedback to optimize dietary and therapeutic protocols based on individual responses and preferences.

Education and Support

- **Nutritional Education**: Provide comprehensive information on the benefits of Raw Veganism, emphasizing its role in enhancing DMSO therapy and supporting overall health.

- **Support Networks**: Facilitate access to dietitians, nutritionists, or Raw Vegan support groups to assist patients in maintaining their dietary regimen alongside DMSO therapy.

Safety Considerations

Nutrient Deficiencies

- **Risk of Deficiencies**: Raw Veganism may lead to deficiencies in essential nutrients such as Vitamin B12, iron, calcium, and omega-3 fatty acids if not properly managed.

- **Mitigation Strategies**: Implement appropriate supplementation and dietary diversification to ensure balanced nutrient intake and prevent deficiencies that could compromise health and therapeutic outcomes.

Gastrointestinal Health

- **High Fiber Intake**: While beneficial for detoxification, excessive fiber intake can cause gastrointestinal discomfort, bloating, or diarrhea, particularly when combined with DMSO's solvent properties.

- **Mitigation Strategies**: Gradually increase fiber intake and ensure adequate hydration to support digestive health and minimize adverse gastrointestinal effects.

Allergic Reactions and Sensitivities

- **Food Allergies**: Patients may have allergies or sensitivities to certain raw plant foods, which can lead to adverse reactions when combined with DMSO therapy.

- **Mitigation Strategies**: Conduct thorough dietary assessments to identify and exclude allergenic foods, and monitor for any signs of allergic reactions during therapy.

Interaction with Medications

- **Pharmacokinetic Interactions**: The enhanced absorption properties of DMSO can alter the pharmacokinetics of medications taken alongside DMSO, necessitating careful management.

- **Mitigation Strategies**: Review all medications and supplements with healthcare providers to identify and manage potential interactions, adjusting dosages as necessary to maintain therapeutic efficacy and safety.

Conclusion

Dimethyl sulfoxide (DMSO) stands as a multifaceted compound with a diverse array of therapeutic applications spanning conventional medicine, alternative therapies, and integrative health practices. Its unique physicochemical properties, particularly its ability to act as a potent solvent and enhance cellular permeability, underpin its effectiveness in various medical and therapeutic contexts. From its approved use in treating interstitial cystitis to its experimental applications in pain management, wound healing, and regenerative medicine, DMSO offers significant potential to address complex health challenges.

The integration of DMSO with conventional treatments exemplifies its role as an adjunctive agent that can amplify the efficacy of established therapies through enhanced drug delivery and synergistic biological effects. Concurrently, its adoption within alternative and naturopathic medicine highlights its versatility and alignment with holistic healing principles, where it complements natural therapies and supports the body's intrinsic healing mechanisms.

Moreover, the interplay between DMSO therapy and lifestyle factors, such as diet and physical activity, underscores the importance of a comprehensive approach to health. Anti-inflammatory diets and specific nutritional strategies can enhance the therapeutic outcomes of DMSO, fostering an environment conducive to optimal healing and well-being. This holistic perspective not only maximizes the benefits of DMSO but also emphasizes the interconnectedness of various health determinants.

Despite its promising applications, the utilization of DMSO is accompanied by a spectrum of considerations that necessitate careful deliberation. The identification of contraindications, understanding potential drug interactions, and adhering to best practices in administration are paramount to ensuring patient safety and treatment efficacy. Furthermore, the existing body of scientific evidence, while supportive of certain uses, calls for more rigorous clinical trials and mechanistic studies to fully elucidate the therapeutic potential and optimize the application protocols of DMSO.

Ethical and regulatory aspects also play a critical role in shaping the landscape of DMSO use. Navigating the regulatory frameworks, ensuring the use of pharmaceutical-grade DMSO, and maintaining informed consent are essential components of responsible practice. As research advances, these frameworks may evolve, potentially expanding the approved uses of DMSO and integrating it more seamlessly into mainstream medical practice.

In conclusion, DMSO represents a compound of considerable interest and utility within the medical and therapeutic arenas. Its capacity to enhance treatment modalities, coupled with its inherent anti-inflammatory and analgesic properties, positions it as a valuable tool in both conventional and alternative medicine. However, realizing its full potential requires a balanced approach that prioritizes evidence-based practice, comprehensive patient evaluation, and ongoing research. By fostering collaboration among healthcare providers, researchers, and patients, the medical community can continue to explore and harness the benefits of DMSO, ultimately contributing to more effective and personalized healthcare solutions.

HERE IS YOU FREE GIFT!

SCAN HERE TO DOWNLOAD IT

Made in United States
Troutdale, OR
11/15/2024

24836378R00091